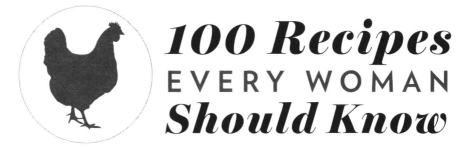

100 Recipes
EVERY WOMAN
Should Know

Cindi Leive

EDITOR-IN-CHIEF

and the Editors of *Glamour*

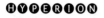

NEW YORK

100 Recipes EVERY WOMAN *Should Know*

Engagement CHICKEN

and 99 Other Fabulous Dishes to Get You Everything You Want in Life

Copyright © 2011 Condé Nast Publications

All rights reserved. No part of this book may be used or reproduced in any manner whatsoever without the written permission of the Publisher. Printed in the United States of America. For information address Hyperion, 114 Fifth Avenue, New York, New York, 10011.

Library of Congress Cataloging-in-Publication Data

100 Recipes Every Woman Should Know : Engagement Chicken and 99 other fabulous dishes to get you everything you want in life : a Glamour cookbook / Cindi Leive, editor-in-chief and the editors of Glamour.
      p.   cm.
  ISBN 978-1-4013-2406-3
  1. Cooking, American.   I. Leive, Cindi.   II. Glamour.   III. Title: 100 Recipes Every Woman Should Know : Engagement chicken and ninety-nine other fabulous dishes to get you everything you want in life.
  TX715.E5677 2010
  641.5973—dc22

                                        2010030780

ISBN 978-1-4013-2406-3

GLAMOUR is a registered trademark of Advance Magazine Publishers Inc.

ENGAGEMENT CHICKEN is a registered trademark of Advance Magazine Publishers Inc.

Hyperion books are available for special promotions and premiums. For details contact the HarperCollins Special Markets Department in the New York office at 212-207-7528, fax 212-207-7222, or email spsales@harper collins.com.

BOOK DESIGN BY SHUBHANI SARKAR

Endpapers
Photographer: Jonny Valiant
Food Stylist: Maggie Ruggiero
Prop Stylist: Jocelyne Beaudoin

First Edition

10   9   8   7   6   5   4   3

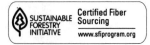

THIS LABEL APPLIES TO TEXT STOCK

We try to produce the most beautiful books possible, and we are also extremely concerned about the impact of our manufacturing process on the forests of the world and the environment as a whole. Accordingly, we've made sure that all of the paper we use has been certified as coming from forests that are managed, to ensure the protection of the people and wildlife dependent upon them.

For any woman
who wants to stir the pot—
in the kitchen, in love, and in *life*.

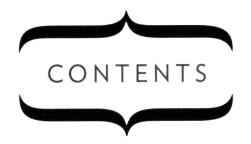

CONTENTS

✳

breakfast & brunch

nibbles

drinks

soups & salads

meat & poultry

seafood

pizza & pasta

meat-free mains

sides

cheap & easy meals

sweets

menus
for occasions big & small

✳

Foreword

WOULD YOU BELIEVE ME IF I TOLD YOU THAT food can get you everything you want in life? Of course not. But it can get you close. That's the message of this book, and if you're rolling your eyes at the idea, well, I was right there with you—until Engagement Chicken persuaded me otherwise. This magical little dish, whose wonderful and romantic story is chronicled in these pages, is responsible for more than 60 engagements so far, and it has turned me into a believer. Not just in the power of a simple roast chicken to make men drop to their knees and propose, but in the power of what we make, and what we eat, to change our moods, our fates, and even, yes, our lives.

Like a lot of women these days, I never really learned to cook. Sure, my mom did it, and very well (flank steak with broccoli was a masterpiece in her hands); and my stepmother, born in Switzerland, is one of the most effortlessly elegant home chefs I know, the kind of woman who can take four eggs and a hunk of cheese and turn it into a fine-dining experience. But growing up, I had more important things to spend my time on. Boys, clothes, plotting my brilliant career—all of it seemed more compelling than anything that might happen in the kitchen.

How naive I was. Only as an adult did I realize—after a few years of trying to subsist on takeout—that cooking is one of life's great pleasures. Even in my shoebox-size apartment,

I discovered that chopping and stirring and mixing and mashing could dissolve all my daily stresses, and the results seemed to work some strange hocus-pocus on the people around me as well. You know the drill: Serve your recently cheated-on best friend homemade muffins and she'll cry—and then realize that she deserves a guy who will take at least as good care of her as you do. Bring the leftover muffins to the office and even Scrooge in the next cubicle will suddenly be verrry, verrry nice. Not that I was instantly good at cooking (it took me far too long to figure out that if you heat the oil too high for the stir-fry, the fire alarm *will* go off, and your cranky super *will* come yell at you). But I liked it, and other people liked it, and I wished I'd spent more time hovering round the stove as a teen, taking notes.

So I turned to cookbooks—and, specifically, to *Glamour* magazine's last cookbook, *Glamour's Gourmet on the Run*, a working-girl bible that offered simple but satisfying recipes for what was then a new generation of time-pressed women. New books were verboten on my starter salary, but I picked up *GOTR* used, and it served me well: The no-cook turkey tonnato charmed the hard-to-charm bridal party of my oldest friend; the filet mignon made a boyfriend I'd offended feel very made-up-to (so much so that we now have two kids); and the pasta-dinner chart page still has my happy tomato splatters on it (we've updated it for you here on page 167).

Today, as the editor of *Glamour*, I'm very pleased that recipes are a staple of the magazine. Our 12 million readers tell us that they cook for all kinds of reasons: because they love it; because they're trying to eat healthfully; because it's so much more affordable than eating out. But many also cook, as I came to, just to see what happens. And sometimes what happens is life-changing. About seven years ago, as you'll read here, we published a recipe for a delicious lemon-infused roast chicken—a recipe one of our own editors had developed, and one of our own staffers had gotten engaged after making. What happened next was a little bit miraculous, and it convinced me that *food gets stuff done.*

Or maybe it's better to say that *you* get stuff done, but food helps. This book, like every recipe that *Glamour* publishes, is written with your crazy life in mind: your schedule (busy), your tastes (diverse), and your kitchen (not staffed with a sous-chef). In the capable hands of cookbook editor Veronica Chambers, every set of instructions was tested by both accomplished home chefs *and* women who say they don't cook, so whatever your kitchen skills, you're covered.

You may be buying this book strictly for the Engagement Chicken and its yummy brand of marital magic. My heart and hopes are with you. But it's just as likely you're not that into chicken, or you don't want to get engaged, or you've already wooed the partner of your dreams. That's fine too. You do want something—probably lots of somethings—out of life. I hope this cookbook helps you get it all, and then some.

Cindi Leive
EDITOR-IN-CHIEF, *Glamour*

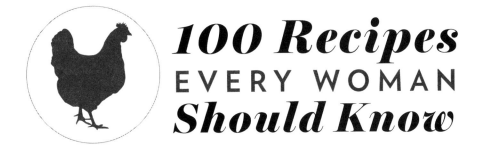

100 Recipes
EVERY WOMAN
Should Know

Introduction

ONCE UPON A TIME, THERE WAS A YOUNG MAGA-zine assistant who loved her boyfriend and imagined that someday in the not too distant future they would get married. One evening, in the kind of flurry of domesticity that even the most modern young woman can experience, she made her boyfriend a classic roast chicken supper, based on a recipe her boss, a *Glamour* editor, had given her. Her boyfriend loved it. He had seconds. He licked his fingers. And shortly thereafter, he proposed.

Naturally, she was overjoyed, and word of her success in the kitchen quickly spread around the office. Recipe tips were shared. Roasting pans were purchased. And, as the staff watched in amazement, *three* assistants in the *Glamour* fashion department were, in short order, engaged.

Just like that, Engagement Chicken was born.

A word about that chicken: It was fabulously simple. Kimberly Bonnell, the then-*Glamour* editor and avid cook who'd developed the recipe, had traveled to Italy and remembered loving the simple roast chicken she ate there because it captured "the real essence of Italian cooking, which was that you did as little as possible to the food." Her recipe, adapted from one by Marcella Hazan, included several tips that made good cooking sense: puncturing the lemons before stuffing them into the chicken so that the deep citrus flavors infused the meat; covering the skin with lemon juice and salt so that it

> 66 *Relationships are complicated. Cooking comes with instructions.* 99
> —MELROSE PLACE

1

engagement CHICKEN
success story

JENNIFER VALE
&
CHRIS GREEN

ST. LOUIS, MO

CHICKEN DATE:
February 14, 2006

ENGAGEMENT DATE:
March 23, 2006

On her first Valentine's Day with boyfriend Chris, then thirty-one—a sweet neighbor who'd wooed her for years by opening doors for her and carrying her shopping bags—*Glamour* reader Jennifer, then thirty-six, decided to make Engagement Chicken. (She swears it wasn't all about the ring; she also just thought it sounded tasty.) "Chris kept talking about how hard the recipe must have been, and I went along for kicks, but really it was so simple," she says. A little more than a month later, on vacation in the Smoky Mountains, Chris got down on one knee in the middle of a snow-covered trail and proposed. When they married the next year, Jennifer made a toast: "If anyone is looking for ideas," she told the crowd, "make that chicken!"

became super-crispy; and most importantly, turning the chicken midway through cooking so that the breast meat, which can get so annoyingly dry in some recipes, stayed just as juicy as the dark pieces. It cooked up impressively, but, notes Bonnell, was a great recipe for "someone who's nervous about being in the kitchen or hasn't cooked a lot. It's really easy to make. Let's not forget about the cook's needs when we're thinking about the guy's needs!"

But back to the weddings. As it turned out, those first three engagements were only the tip of the chicken iceberg. In 2004, *Glamour* published the recipe in the magazine. Almost immediately, the letters started pouring in:

> 66 I made Engagement Chicken for my live-in boyfriend and today, I'm wearing a wedding band. This chicken is serious stuff. But please keep me anonymous—my husband doesn't know that he was reeled in by a chicken. 99

> 66 My boyfriend and I had looked at rings, but he hadn't proposed. I decided to make Engagement Chicken after hearing it had become a superstition for girls everywhere. I joked to him that maybe this would speed things along—and sure enough, right after dinner, he was down on one knee. Boy, did my Engagement Chicken work—thanks, *Glamour!* 99

> 66 You don't even have to *make* the chicken for it to work. I bought all the ingredients, and while they were sitting in my kitchen, he dragged me into the bedroom (which was full of candles), got down on both knees, and asked me to marry him. 99

Sometimes the proposals were instantaneous, as if the chicken had a secret "marry-me-let's-spend-the-rest-of-our-lives-together" chemical that kicked in right away, the same way tryptophan can make you want to nap after a big turkey dinner. And, some letter-writers noted, the bride didn't even have to be the one cooking. Nicole Ives, then twenty-five, of Cooperstown, NY, had been dating her boyfriend Anthony Suhadolnik, then twenty-three, for exactly a year and ten days (not that she'd been counting!) when they visited Nicole's pal Casey Ringeisen in Washington, DC, for the weekend. The night before they arrived, Casey had made Engagement Chicken for *her* boyfriend, hoping that he would propose (which, alas, he didn't). She used the leftovers to make chicken-salad sandwiches for Nicole and Anthony before the couple went sightseeing. Anthony strangely insisted they take a walk to the Washington Monument, despite the pouring rain. You guessed it: He needed a romantic proposal spot. Chicken strikes again! (Back home, Casey pulled out her *Glamour* clipping and told Nicole and Anthony what she'd served them.) Says Casey, "I guess your Engagement Chicken does seal the deal, just not always for the person who cooks it!"

Oh, and if you're not even romantically involved with the guy yet? Engagement Chicken can fix that too. One letter-writer, Angela Warren, then twenty-six, of Cedar Rapids, Iowa, had offered to cook dinner for a man she was just friends with, Jason Roorda, then twenty-four, and pulled the recipe from *Glamour* because it looked like a good dinner-party dish. "I had no hidden agenda," she says. "I simply wanted to try it out." The chicken was a huge hit and, after dinner that night, out of nowhere, Jason kissed Angela. A month and a half later, they were engaged. "To this day, the chicken is still one of Jason's absolute favorites," Angela says. "What's amazing to me is that the recipe was powerful enough to make a man I never even dated propose!"

Before we knew it, the chicken had made national news. "Want a Rock? Get Your Chicken On," read one Fox News

engagement CHICKEN *success story*

PAULA VÁSQUEZ
&
BRANDON GALLION
PORTLAND, OR

CHICKEN DATE:
February 20, 2010

ENGAGEMENT DATE:
March 6, 2010

It's true: Engagement Chicken works even if you don't make it yourself! See if you can follow this twisted tale. When Sheri, a friend of Brandon's mother, invited him and girlfriend Paula to dinner, the couple thought it was just to welcome them to town; they'd recently moved to Portland. But Sheri had "read about a chicken recipe with special marriage-making powers," she says. "I thought I'd see if it worked." And sure enough, a few weeks later, Brandon, then twenty-four, and Paula, then twenty-three, were out walking their dogs when he turned to her and said, "I have a question for you." (You know the rest.) As soon as Brandon's mother e-mailed the news to all her girlfriends, Sheri came clean and forwarded the recipe to all the moms in the group—so they could get *their* kids married off too. Make it "because it is delicious and easy," she wrote, "but be careful who you serve it to!"

engagement
CHICKEN
success story

AMBER FRICKE
&
MARK BENTOSKI

HAMPTON, VA

CHICKEN DATE:
July 16, 2009

ENGAGEMENT DATE:
September 5, 2009

One hot summer day, Amber, then twenty-eight, left work early to make Engagement Chicken for her boyfriend of nearly two years, Mark. "I wanted good marriage karma," she says—and she was hoping the chicken might jolt him into action. When Mark, then thirty-two, came home, he was suspicious: "You're baking a chicken on a work night?" he asked. But he enjoyed his dinner and, a few months later, asked Amber on a motorcycle trip. Each time they pulled over to take pictures of the gorgeous views, she'd think, This is it! "I'd take my helmet off, fluff my hair, and... nothing." Finally, watching the sunset on a mountainside, Mark said the words every woman wants to hear: "I'd get down on one knee, but I don't want to fall off this cliff."

headline. "Engagement Chicken: A Magical Food That Causes Marriage," blared a blog. *Glamour* editors prepared the meal live on the *Today* show, and chef Ina Garten cooked up her own delicious version on her *Barefoot Contessa* TV program. In her most recent cookbook, *How Easy Is That?* she dedicates the chicken to her husband, Jeffrey, writing, "Recently, I met some beautiful young women from *Glamour* magazine. They make a roast chicken they call 'Engagement Chicken' because every time one of them makes it for her boyfriend, she gets engaged! How wonderful is that? That's the best reason I ever heard to make a roast chicken!"

Along the way, the requests from readers started mounting: "I NEED to make this!" e-mailed one woman. "Please send the recipe!!" Mothers—you know mothers!—even called the office asking if they could have the recipe for their daughters. One commenter on glamour.com, preparing to cook her bird, posted this question: "Was just wondering if the ring would be bigger if I cooked a turkey . . . or if a Cornish hen would get me a smaller ring?" (Don't worry. She was kidding. "Either way, I love him. . . . I don't really need a ring at all," she promised.)

One morning, radio host Howard Stern, unaware of the dish's name or purpose, waxed poetic on air about the amazing meal he'd been served the night before by then-girlfriend Beth Ostrosky. When a female listener phoned in to say the dish sounded suspiciously like the Engagement Chicken she'd read about in *Glamour*, Howard called Beth at home on the air, woke her up, and made her answer for herself. She fessed up, and later, after Stern had (of course!) proposed, she talked about Engagement Chicken on the *Rachael Ray* show. "I recommend it for any girl out there," she has said.

So why does the chicken work? We've all heard the cliché "the way to a man's heart is through his stomach," or, as Honoré de Balzac put it back in the nineteenth century, "Men become passionately attached to women who know how to cosset them with delicate tidbits." But why *this* delicate tidbit in particular and not, say, eggplant parm or ham sandwiches?

Kimberly Bonnell thinks she knows. The chicken, she realized soon after devising the recipe, was guaranteed guy-friendly: familiar but different, fancier than everyday chicken but not off-puttingly strange or fussy. In that sense, Engagement Chicken is a show-them-the-love dish, not a show-them-the-sweat-on-your-brow one. You planned to make a nice roast chicken dinner. You went to the market, did some prep work, minded the oven, and prepared some sides. It is not the kind of dish that says "I took the day off from work and went to twelve different markets to get all of these exotic ingredients to make you lobster Newburg and salmon terrine and apricot soufflé. Do you like it? Huh? Huh? Do you?" No one wants *that*. Engagement Chicken is the culinary equivalent of a perfect tee and jeans: lived in, gorgeous, and not trying too hard.

Besides, roast chicken is comforting: It sends the signal that the cook can take care of the people she is close to. For decades Pillsbury ran a campaign that said, "Nothin' says lovin' like something from the oven." It sounds ridiculously retro, but frankly, it's true. Roast chicken is old-school—and an unexpected thing to find young women, raised on the microwave and the takeout menu, whipping up. "A roast chicken is a meal for two," points out Laura Shapiro, a food historian and author of *Perfection Salad: Women and Cooking at the Turn of the Century.* "It's a choice that's very intimate."

Many of the women who made Engagement Chicken readily acknowledged that it was out of character for them to do *anything* domestic. Exhibit A: Glamour.com editor Lindsey Unterberger, then twenty-five, who dubbed herself "Engagement Chick" after she decided to prepare the meal for her boyfriend Aaron Perlstein, then twenty-six. "What is a roasting pan?" she blogged, not entirely exaggerating. "OMG, WTF is a

---

engagement CHICKEN *success story*

HOLLY LEAHY & JEREMY KIJOWSKI

ST. LOUIS, MO

CHICKEN DATE:
December 19, 2008

ENGAGEMENT DATE:
December 19, 2008 (yup, same night!)

Jeremy, then twenty-five, had loved Holly, then twenty-six, since they'd met. And finally, two and a half years after that, she was ready for a lifelong commitment. So she decided their typical Friday date night was about to get a major upgrade from movies and popcorn. Unfortunately, the recipe that she'd cut out from *Glamour* didn't seem like an instant hit. "He only had a few bites," remembers Holly. Turns out it wasn't her meal that had turned his stomach—it was nerves! Shortly after picking at his food, Jeremy said he was going to get dessert. He returned with a cake box, and when Holly opened it, she found a velvet ring case nestled inside. Jeremy swears the menu was a coincidence and that he was going to ask all along. But, says Holly, "*I* know—it was the chicken!"

engagement CHICKEN
success story

MADELEINE MAYHER
&
BRIAN VAN ALMEN

BAY VILLAGE, OH

CHICKEN DATE:
October 21, 2004

ENGAGEMENT DATE:
October 21, 2004 (that same night!)

For her guy's twenty-sixth birthday, Madeleine, then twenty-three, decided to try *Glamour*'s Engagement Chicken recipe—no small endeavor considering she'd been a vegetarian for ten years and had only just started eating chicken again. Brian loved his meal and after the dinner, handed the cook a gift: a pair of slippers...with an engagement ring nestled inside. She immediately said yes and, later that night "told him that he wasn't going to believe what I'd cooked him for dinner. When I revealed the name of the chicken, he laughed and said: 'It really works!'" And it did: not just for Madeleine but for her younger sister, too, who, hearing of her sister's success, made the same recipe for *her* boyfriend—and also got engaged.

giblet? Can I hire someone to do this for me? God, this is going to be a DISASTER." But she pulled it off, and Aaron (now her husband) was, frankly, floored. "I would have to say the chicken was memorable because it was one of the first non-mac-and-cheese dishes I'd ever seen Lindsey cook!" he says now.

And then there's Karie Anderson—*so* not a chef—who burned her hand and overcooked the meat but managed to make the *Glamour* staff cry with her touching story. Karie and her boyfriend Kyle John were living in young, normal-couple bliss in San Diego when Kyle was diagnosed with Ewing's sarcoma, a rare type of bone cancer. In a few months' time, "he went from being this energetic soccer player type to barely being able to walk," Karie says. Kyle lost all of his thick curly hair, needed round-the-clock care, and one day told Karie, "If you want to leave me, I'll understand." Karie didn't want to leave him. She wanted to be with him for as long as she could. So she made Kyle Engagement Chicken.

Like we said, the girl isn't getting her own cooking show anytime soon, but Kyle was impressed with her efforts. "Of all the meals, why did you decide to bake a chicken?" he asked. Karie, then twenty-seven, just shrugged. A few weeks later, Kyle, then twenty-seven, made his bittersweet proposal. "I'm probably not going to get better," he told Karie. "If I die, I want you to be more than a girlfriend. I want you to be my wife."

Less than a month afterward, the couple exchanged vows in front of family and friends. Kyle was frail, barely able to stand for photos. After his death, Karie wrote to us to say thank you. The recipe, she felt, made her take action when she didn't have time to waste. "I'm still grieving," she says. "But I'm lucky because I know what true love is. I had it with him."

Karie's letter made us all pause, and think about love, life, and what really matters.

Chicken can be as deep as you want it to be.

＊

THAT'S WHAT THIS BOOK IS ALL ABOUT: SQUEEZING EVERY drop of juice out of your sweet life. Of course, there's more to that life than weddings. And there's more—*much* more—than Engagement Chicken to this cookbook. It's filled with ninety-nine of *Glamour*'s other most-loved, best-reviewed recipes, all designed to get you exactly what you want, exactly when you want it. If you're not *quite* ready for Engagement Chicken, there's Instant Seduction Pork Chops (page 117)—which amazingly don't even require a pan, so you can skip the cleanup and get to the, um, dessert; and, for the next morning, He Stayed Over Omelet, page 23 (designed to be made with whatever's in your fridge, so no one has to go out to shop in their skivvies). To solve any cooking-for-a-crowd situation, there's It's Almost Payday Chili (page 204) and BFF Birthday Cake (page 219). Getting home late after work? Try making Who Calls a Meeting at 5:00 P.M.? Stir-Fry (page 175) or, perhaps, Forget the Mistake You Made at Work Margarita, page 67 (we've all been there!). Meantime, there's Let's Make a Baby Pasta (page 157), No Guy Required Grilled Steak (page 111), Bribe a Kid Brownies (page 233), and Prove to Mom You're Not Going to Starve Meat Loaf (page 107)—which, incidentally, works just as well at reassuring your parents when you're forty-five as when you're twenty-two. And throughout you'll find easy, quick meals to make for when it's just you, too. Because, repeat after us: Cereal isn't dinner!

There are many things in life that will make you feel as if you've arrived, from owning your first grown-up designer handbag to owning your own home. But there is no greater and more easily attainable upgrade than learning how to cook for yourself. It has the seemingly contradictory effect of saving you money and making you feel rich. Whether you've picked this book up at the beginning of your culinary adventure, or

> 66 *One cannot think well, love well, sleep well, if one has not dined well.*99
>
> —VIRGINIA WOOLF, *A ROOM OF ONE'S OWN*

engagement
CHICKEN
success story

KELLY PRICE
&
BRANDON GEYER

SAN ANTONIO, TX

CHICKEN DATE:
December 20, 2009

ENGAGEMENT DATE:
December 20, 2009

Engagement Chicken isn't just for ladies—men, too, have given the recipe a whirl. Though normally not one to cook, Brandon, then twenty-six, decided to make Engagement Chicken for his girlfriend Kelly, then twenty-five, after hearing Howard Stern talk about it on air. It was Sunday, so he had an entire day off from work to set the scene for his proposal: He cleaned the house, set the table, and prepped the chicken. "Hopefully, I'll only have to make this recipe once," he told his family (who were rooting for them) on the phone. No worries: Kelly loved the chicken…and said yes to the ring.

you are a confident home cook looking to expand your repertoire, the recipes featured here are designed to help you cook with passion and persuasion. We've written all of them with your real life and real needs in mind. Among the assumptions we're making:

- You probably don't want recipes that call for ingredients that can only be ordered from exotic Web sites with two weeks' shipping time. (Who plans that far ahead?) Almost everything on our ingredient lists can be found at your local supermarket.

- There will be some nights when you are feeling ambitious in the kitchen (in which case, we'd like to recommend Can We Talk? Crab Cakes, page 135) and others when you just want to get on the couch in front of *Glee* as quickly as possible (hello, Lazy Day Frittata, page 211).

- You may or may not own a food processor or a spice mill (all optional in preparing most of our dishes), but you most certainly do *not* have your own personal baguette-making machine, and you think anyone who does should be committed.

Throughout the book you'll see a three-stiletto key—explained on page 15—to help you judge a recipe's level of difficulty. Most dishes are one- and two-stiletto jobs, but even the three-stiletto numbers are easy to master. Because whether you're a novice or an expert, cooking should never be intimidating—and it should always be *fun*.

✻

IN PUTTING THIS COOKBOOK TOGETHER, WE'VE TAKEN A lot of inspiration and ideas from *you*. (Thanks for that!) Many of you have asked what the vegetarian equivalent of Engagement Chicken is, so we spent months cooking up our favorite meatless dishes and ultimately settled on a delicious paella, especially impressive when served steamy, straight out of the pan. It's part of a whole chapter on Meat-Free Mains; don't miss Meatless Monday Portobello Burgers (page 177), inspired by designer Stella McCartney, who shared this astounding statistic with us: If every American skipped one meal of chicken a week, it would be the energy-saving equivalent of taking *half a million* cars off the road. Many of you have taken up cooking as a way to eat affordably—so we've created a Cheap and Easy Meals chapter, full of recipes that taste much richer than they cost. (The Pauper's Fish Feast, page 206, made with wallet-friendly tilapia, is an especially nice discovery.) And while no cookbook is truly great without a little butter, sometimes you just want something good and healthy. Your girlfriends will rave over your No-Fail Kale Salad (page 89), and I Got Thinner Eating Pasta (page 158) is not a joke. It's real, and it's spectacular.

We've also included a section of menus, to make cooking for life's trickiest occasions a little less so. There's an Engagement Chicken dinner menu, of course—and it's romantic. But there's also a lower-key I Like You Enough to Cook Dinner menu for when you're first getting to know a guy; and, for the Super Bowl or the season finale of *Mad Men*, a Don't Block the TV Dinner Party. Finally, there's a suggested pantry list of all the little essentials that clever cooks have on hand: Stock your cabinets with them and you'll always have something to make. Many, like Arborio rice and cans of San Marzano tomatoes, will last you months and months.

✻

IT IS AN ICONIC MOMENT IN TELEVISION: THE GREAT JULIA
Child drops a piece of potato pancake, then cheerfully picks

---

engagement
CHICKEN
success story

NICOLE WASSON
&
DAVE SZCZEPANSKI
WATERFORD, MI

CHICKEN DATE:
February 15, 2004

ENGAGEMENT DATE:
February 21, 2004

Never the timid type, Nicole, then thirty, had openly talked about wanting to get engaged, and had even showed her boyfriend, Dave, then twenty-nine, pictures of rings she liked. When Valentine's Day came, she cranked it up a notch and made the chicken. "I don't usually cook," she notes—Dave does that—"so if I can make this recipe, anyone can!" The following Friday, Dave called Nicole into the bedroom—where she found him on bended knee, surrounded by rose petals and candles, with Sarah McLachlan's "Ice Cream" playing on the stereo. (You know: "Your love is better than ice cream." This guy is *good*!) Dave disputes Engagement Chicken's role in the proposal, saying he was going to get around to it anyway, but Nicole feels otherwise: "You ate the chicken, and I got the ring!" she says. "That's what matters."

engagement
CHICKEN
success story

PAULA DITTEON
&
JOSH SCHULTZ

HUNTSVILLE, AL

CHICKEN DATE:
October 10, 2009

ENGAGEMENT DATE:
October 25, 2009

"We're both picky eaters," Paula, then twenty-five, says, so when she was hunting for a new, slightly more adventurous recipe to make for her boyfriend of two years, this one-step-up-from-basic chicken sounded perfect. And although Josh, then twenty-nine, *loved* the meal, he didn't seem particularly matrimonial after eating it. But behold: Two weeks later, the couple was lying on the kitchen floor using an air pressure gun to do some home remodeling, when Josh turned to Paula and asked, out of nowhere, "Will you marry me?" Paula said yes (and no one was injured!). "I love this chicken," says Paula, "because now there's a way to drop a hint without being blatant."

it up and puts it back in the pan. "If you're alone in your kitchen, who's going to see?" she trills, by which she means your culinary mishaps are your own.

Heretical as it may sound, we've written this cookbook with quite the opposite thought in mind. You need never feel alone in your kitchen, because 12 million *Glamour* readers—and we, the editors—are there with you as sous-chefs, cheering you on in the kitchen and in life. We can't wait to hear about your successes, your big nights, your little triumphs, and yes—your engagements.

As the great Rosalind Russell said in *Auntie Mame,* "Life is a banquet." Here's what to serve at yours.

P.S. If you do make Engagement Chicken and get engaged (or make any of the other recipes in this book with happy results), please e-mail us at: engagementchicks@glamour.com. We can't wait to hear from you.

The Engagement Chicken Hall of Fame (So Far)

We've heard from sixty-plus women who've gotten married (or plan to) after making our famous bird. Meet just a few of the happy couples.

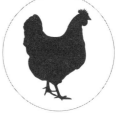

ANN WRIGHT
&
MICHAEL DRAPER

DAVISON, MI

*

WEDDING DATE:
April 3, 2004

RACHEL DESTEFANO
&
MATTHEW BAUMAN

MOUNT JULIET, TN

*

WEDDING DATE:
August 7, 2005

TORI ADKINS
&
JASON SADNICK

LA MOILLE, IL

*

WEDDING DATE:
April 29, 2006

ANGELA WARREN
&
JASON ROORDA

CEDAR RAPIDS, IA

*

WEDDING DATE:
September 16, 2006

SARAH MOZELLE
&
EN KARAKOTSIOS

SAN JOSE, CA

*

WEDDING DATE:
August 21, 2004

MADELEINE MAYHER
&
BRIAN VAN ALMEN

BAY VILLAGE, OH

*

WEDDING DATE:
August 12, 2005

BELLA
&
MIKE

CHICAGO, IL

*

WEDDING DATE:
July 18, 2006

JENNIFER VALE
&
CHRIS GREEN

ST. LOUIS, MO

*

WEDDING DATE:
June 1, 2007

LAURA WHEELER
&
TOM WHEELER

ST. LOUIS, MO

*

WEDDING DATE:
November 20, 2004

CATHIE MILLER
&
GREGG BAILEY

DORCHESTER, MA

*

WEDDING DATE:
September 24, 2005

NAOMI REIDNAUER
&
DARRELL MOSHER

GREENEVILLE, TN

*

WEDDING DATE:
September 8, 2006

BRIDGETTE MARTIN
&
COLEY O'DELL

KNOXVILLE, TN

*

WEDDING DATE:
November 3, 2007

NICOLE WASSON
&
AVE SZCZEPANSKI

WATERFORD, MI

*

WEDDING DATE:
July 30, 2005

JENNIFER O'SHIELDS
&
MICHAEL DRAPER

LEXINGTON, SC

*

WEDDING DATE:
October 8, 2005

DAWN LAWKOWSKI
&
JAMES KELLER

CHICAGO, IL

*

WEDDING DATE:
September 10, 2006

DORIS HERNANDEZ
&
KARL MYERS

BROOKLYN, NY

*

WEDDING DATE:
June 14, 2008

KARIE ANDERSON
&
R. KYLE JOHN III

SAN DIEGO, CA

*

WEDDING DATE:
June 21, 2008

BETH OSTROSKY
&
HOWARD STERN

NEW YORK, NY

*

WEDDING DATE:
October 3, 2008

REBECCA ZENS
&
JOHN BOHN

RACINE, WI

*

WEDDING DATE:
July 18, 2009

LINDSAY WEBSTER
&
STEVE NADRAMIA

SELDEN, NY

*

WEDDING DATE:
August 22, 2009

NICOLE IVES
&
ANTHONY SUHADOLNIK

COOPERSTOWN, NY

*

WEDDING DATE:
September 5, 2009

SAMANTHA BERRY
&
SEÁN NUTLEY

VANCOUVER, BC

*

WEDDING DATE:
September 12, 2009

DONNA RZYMOWSKI
&
DOMINIC CHIOVARI

WAUCONDA, IL

*

WEDDING DATE:
October 17, 2009

ASHLEY LANNING
&
DAVID CRIMMINS

MUSCATINE, IA

*

WEDDING DATE:
November 2, 2009

MALLORY SHARP
&
GREG EVANS

OKLAHOMA CITY, OK

*

WEDDING DATE:
February 6, 2010

NANCY COLLINS
&
GREG GELPI

ATLANTA, GA

*

WEDDING DATE:
March 13, 2010

AMELIA COATES
&
DANNY COATES

WEST GROVE, PA

*

WEDDING DATE:
April 2, 2010

HOLLY LEAHY
&
JEREMY KIJOWSKI

ST. LOUIS, MO

*

WEDDING DATE:
April 17, 2010

AMBER FRICKE
&
MARK BENTOSKI

HAMPTON, VA

*

WEDDING DATE:
May 8, 2010

KIMBERLY STEENO
&
JASON DECUR

GREEN BAY, WI

*

WEDDING DATE:
May 15, 2010

EMILY QUAIL
&
JOSH BURWELL

BETHESDA, MD

*

WEDDING DATE:
May 22, 2010

ROSARIO ARAGUAS
&
WESLEY LAVOIE

EL CENTRO, CA

*

WEDDING DATE:
May 29, 2010

DESIREE LUECK
&
SHANE LUND

VICTORVILLE, CA

*

WEDDING DATE:
June 5, 2010

MANDY SPENCER
&
DEREK CONLIN

RALEIGH, NC

*

WEDDING DATE:
June 26, 2010

ALYSSA LOFGREN
&
MATT CURRAN

RESEDA, CA

*

WEDDING DATE:
August 7, 2010

LINDSEY UNTERBERGER
&
AARON PERLSTEIN

NEW YORK, NY

*

WEDDING DATE:
August 14, 2010

PAULA DITTEON
&
JOSH SCHULTZ

HUNTSVILLE, AL

*

WEDDING DATE:
August 14, 2010

MELISSA MARTY
&
DAVID SNYDER

ASHLAND, OH

*

WEDDING DATE:
May 29, 2011

AMANDA GREENSPAN
&
COREY STEVENS

MIDDLETOWN, RI

*

WEDDING DATE:
July 30, 2011

KIM WILSON
&
TRAVIS GUILEY

SANTA CRUZ, CA

*

WEDDING DATE:
September 17, 2011

PAULA VÁSQUEZ
&
BRANDON GALLION

PORTLAND, OR

*

WEDDING DATE:
September 12, 2010

IRENE MAYHER
&
DAVE STRACHAN

CLEVELAND HEIGHTS, OH

*

WEDDING DATE:
July 30, 2011

KELLY PRICE
&
BRANDON GEYER

SAN ANTONIO, TX

*

WEDDING DATE:
September 10, 2011

TANIA KATHERINE
&
MICHAEL W.

CINCINNATI, OH

*

WEDDING DATE:
October 2011

BETSY KELLY
&
RUSSELL TURLEY

JACKSON, MS

*

WEDDING DATE:
March 5, 2011

RACHEL BAUER
&
RICHARD RACZOK

FREMONT, MI

*

WEDDING DATE:
July 30, 2011

ALYSSA GUGLIOTTI
&
LYLE STEVENS

BOSTON, MA

*

WEDDING DATE:
September 10, 2011

Just How Easy Is Each Recipe?

To guide you through the kitchen skills it takes to make the dishes in this cook-book, we've devised a handy stiletto key. (What? You were expecting spatu-las?) Here's how our three-stiletto rating system breaks down:

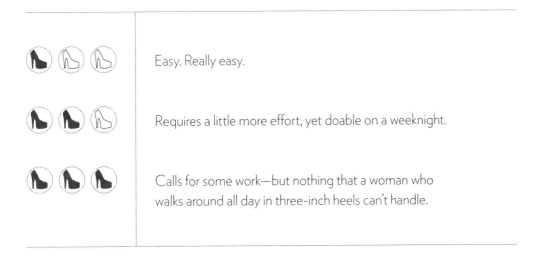

	Easy. Really easy.
	Requires a little more effort, yet doable on a weeknight.
	Calls for some work—but nothing that a woman who walks around all day in three-inch heels can't handle.

engagement
CHICKEN

Engagement Chicken

Roast Chicken with Lemon and Herbs

Serves 2 to 4

1 whole chicken (approximately
  4 pounds)
½ cup fresh lemon juice, plus 3 whole
  lemons—including 1 sliced for garnish
1 tablespoon kosher or coarse sea salt
½ teaspoon freshly ground pepper
Fresh herbs for garnish (4 rosemary
  sprigs, 4 sage sprigs, 8 thyme sprigs,
  and 1 bunch flat-leaf parsley)

Here it is: the recipe that started it all. And once you've made it, you'll know why: It serves up the kind of home-cooked goodness that no restaurant meal can top. The chicken's crispy skin is drenched in herb-infused juices (don't forget to pour the pan drippings back over the chicken before serving or, alternately, to drizzle them over individual pieces on the plate), and the trick of turning the chicken 15 minutes into cooking keeps the meat uniquely moist.

We've suggested a complete menu on page 245, but honestly, any simple sides will work with a main course this splendid. You can go with either white wine (in which case a Riesling would be nice) or red (try pinot noir). Happy cooking—and an even happier future to you and the lucky person you've deemed worthy of this dish.

Oh, and if you have commitment issues? Skip to the next section, woman! This bird means business.

1. Position an oven rack in the upper third of the oven and preheat the oven to 400°F. Remove the giblets from the chicken, wash the chicken inside and out with cold water, then let the chicken drain, cavity down, in a colander for 2 minutes.

2. Pat the chicken dry with paper towels. Place the chicken breast-side down in a medium roasting pan fitted with a rack and pour the lemon juice all over the chicken, both inside and out. Season the chicken all over with salt and pepper inside and out.

[CONTINUED]

3. Prick 2 whole lemons three times each in three different places with a fork and place them deep inside the cavity. Chicken cavity size may vary, so if one lemon is partly sticking out, that's fine. (Tip: If the lemons are stiff, roll them on the countertop with your palm before pricking to get the juices flowing.)

4. Put the chicken in the oven, lower the oven temperature to 350°F, and roast, uncovered, for 15 minutes.

5. Remove the roasting pan from the oven. Using tongs or two wooden spoons, turn the chicken breast-side up. Insert a meat thermometer in the thigh, and return the chicken to the oven and roast for about 1 hour to 1 hour and 15 minutes or until the meat thermometer reads 180°F and the juices run clear when the thigh is pricked with a fork. Continue roasting if necessary. Keep in mind that cooking times in different ovens vary; roasting a chicken at 350°F takes approximately 18–20 minutes per pound, plus an additional 15 minutes.

6. Let the chicken rest for 10 minutes before carving. And here's the secret: Pour the juices from the roasting pan on top of the sliced chicken—this is the "marry me juice." Garnish with fresh herbs and lemon slices.

glamour girl tip

Carving a bird takes a lot of practice, so don't expect it to be perfect on your first try. The most important thing is to have a sharp knife (preferably one made specifically for carving). Start by slicing the breasts, removing as much meat as possible, and then remove the legs and the wings (using kitchen shears works well too). Don't worry if it looks messy; it will taste just as good!

breakfast

&

brunch

He Stayed Over Omelet

Omelet with Fresh Greens, Cherry Tomatoes, and Parmesan Cheese

He's cute. And smart. And funny. And you're *very* glad he stayed the night. No need to break the spell by going out for brunch. This easy omelet is delicious with whatever you find hiding in your fridge. Think he might be staying over a lot? We won't judge. Just keep precooked sausage on hand and your produce drawer filled.

Serves 2

1 or 2 tablespoons butter
½ cup chopped mushrooms (optional)
4 large eggs, lightly beaten
2 tablespoons half-and-half
Salt and freshly ground pepper
¼ cup quartered cherry tomatoes
2 tablespoons chopped fresh spinach (basil or arugula works fine too); if using frozen spinach, thaw it first, then drain it
¼ cup chopped ham, precooked sausage (such as chorizo), smoked sausage, or sausage patties (optional)
¼ cup freshly grated Parmigiano-Reggiano cheese

1. Preheat the broiler. If using mushrooms, melt 1 tablespoon butter in a small skillet and add the mushrooms. Sauté, stirring a few times, until softened, about 2 minutes. Set aside.

2. In a medium bowl, whisk the eggs with half-and-half and a pinch each of salt and pepper.

3. In a medium ovenproof skillet (it *must* be ovenproof), melt 1 tablespoon butter over moderately low heat. Pour the egg mixture into the skillet and cook without stirring, until the eggs begin to set, about 2 minutes. Scatter the tomatoes and greens over the eggs along with the meat and mushrooms, if using. Cook, without stirring, until the eggs are almost completely set, about 3 minutes longer.

4. Sprinkle the cheese on top of the eggs, then slide the skillet under the broiler. Broil until the omelet is golden and set, about 2 minutes. Remove from the broiler.

5. Using a spatula, fold the omelet over and slide it onto a plate. Serve.

Lap of Luxury Eggs with Absolutely Perfect Bacon

An Extra-Soft, Slow-Cooked Scramble and Crisp, Oven-Cooked Bacon

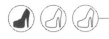

Serves 2

5 large eggs
Salt and freshly ground pepper
1½ tablespoons butter

For *Glamour* assistant editor Carly Suber, making breakfast used to consist of pouring milk into a bowl of Lucky Charms. And while she has mastered this culinary skill, for years it was pretty much the only one she had. Now, thanks to this recipe, she can boast another, infinitely more impressive dish in her repertoire: these perfect creamy eggs, lovely on their own or company-ready when mixed with tomatoes and basil or smoked salmon.

The bacon is more than a side and is really a star in its own right. This ingenious, in-the-oven Southern cooking technique delivers diner-style crispness without the splattery mess. The brown sugar "candies" the bacon, making it even more decadent. Using the oven adds a few minutes to the cooking time, but cleanup is a cinch.

AN EXTRA-SOFT, SLOW-COOKED SCRAMBLE

1. In a medium bowl, whisk eggs with a pinch each of salt and pepper. In a large skillet, melt the butter over moderate heat, tilting to coat the skillet. Turn the heat down to low. Add the eggs and cook, stirring frequently but gently with a wooden spoon, until the eggs turn creamy and pale yellow, about 10 minutes. (Keep the heat as low as it can go without turning off the flame. The egg mixture should get a little lumpy, but it shouldn't stick to the bottom; if it does, keep stirring with one hand but remove the skillet from the stovetop with the other to let it cool a few moments before returning it to the heat.)

2. Continue to cook, breaking up any lumps with the wooden spoon, until soft curds form, as much as 5 to 10 minutes longer (they should still be moist). Remove from the heat *before* the eggs look completely done, since they'll keep cooking for a bit afterward. Continue to stir until cooked through. Transfer to plates and serve right away.

VARIATION 1: WITH TOMATO AND BASIL

Once the eggs have started to form soft curds, stir in the tomato and basil. Serve.

½ cup diced tomato
1 tablespoon chopped fresh basil

VARIATION 2: WITH SMOKED SALMON

Once the eggs have started to form soft curds, stir in the smoked salmon and cream cheese. Garnish the eggs with fresh chives and serve.

A few slices of smoked salmon, diced
1 tablespoon cream cheese
1 tablespoon chopped fresh chives

CRISP, OVEN-COOKED BACON

1. Preheat the oven to 400°F.

2. Line a large, rimmed baking sheet with foil (for easy cleanup), then place a rack over it and lay the bacon on top. For a sweet and savory twist, sprinkle the bacon lightly with brown sugar before baking.

Thickly sliced bacon
  (2 or 3 slices per person)
Brown sugar, for sprinkling (optional)

3. Cook the bacon in the oven for 20 to 25 minutes, or until crispy. (Thinner bacon may take a little less time.) Let cool slightly before serving.

Big Day Steak and Eggs

Sirloin Steak with Fried Eggs and Tomatoes

Serves 2

Two 6- to 8-ounce sirloin steaks,
  each about 1 inch thick
3 tablespoons olive oil
Salt and freshly ground pepper
1 tablespoon minced chives

Are *Glamour*'s health editors suggesting you plow through a huge hunk of sirloin for breakfast every day? No. But for special mornings, this hungry-woman meal satisfies like nothing else. Amanda Grooms West, beauty researcher and resident steak-and-eggs expert, says the genius egg-frying method is the trick. To cook them flawlessly sunny-side up, with fully-cooked whites and oozy yolks, crack the eggs into a hot pan, then almost immediately turn the heat way down. When they're cooked to perfection (and they will be), carefully slide the eggs onto the plate—the generous amount of butter in the recipe makes this easy. Don't sweat the calorie wallop: This special treat almost guarantees you'll want a light lunch.

SIRLOIN STEAK

1. Preheat the oven to 350°F. Heat a medium-size ovenproof skillet over moderate heat for about 5 minutes. Meanwhile, pat the steaks dry with paper towels. Rub the steaks with 2 tablespoons olive oil, and season generously with salt and pepper. Turn the heat up to high and add the remaining 1 tablespoon oil to the skillet. Carefully place the steaks in the skillet (the oil may splatter). Cook, turning once, until browned but still only partially cooked within, about 5 minutes total.

2. Transfer the skillet to the oven and cook the steaks, turning once, about 4 minutes longer, until medium-rare to

medium. (Make sure to use an oven mitt when removing the skillet from the oven; the handle will be hot.)

3. Put the steaks on a plate or cutting board, cover with aluminum foil, and let rest for 10 minutes. Meanwhile, prepare the fried eggs and tomatoes (recipes follow).

4. To serve, place 2 fried eggs on each plate, along with a few slices of cooked tomato. Cut the steaks into thick slices on the diagonal (at a 45-degree angle to the edge of the steak, to break up the grain so you end up with more tender slices). Then arrange between the two plates. Garnish with chopped chives and serve immediately.

FRIED EGGS

1. Heat a medium or large skillet, ideally nonstick, over moderate heat. After a minute, add the butter, and make sure it coats the pan as it's melting. In about another minute, after the foam dies down, crack the eggs into the pan. As soon as the whites have turned opaque (in about 45 seconds to 1 minute), turn the heat down to low.

2. Season the eggs with salt and pepper. Cook until the whites are firm and the yolks are runny. Slide eggs onto plates.

2 tablespoons butter
4 large eggs
Salt and freshly ground pepper

TOMATOES

In the same skillet as the eggs, heat the butter or olive oil over moderate heat. Add the tomato slices. Season them with salt and pepper, and cook for 2 minutes, until softened.

1 tablespoon butter or olive oil
1 tomato, cut into 1-inch-thick slices
Salt and freshly ground pepper

Western-Movie Migas

Tex-Mex–Style Scrambled Eggs with Crunchy Tortilla Strips

Serves 4

⅓ cup vegetable oil

Three 6-inch corn tortillas, sliced into
    thin strips

1 teaspoon salt

1 medium onion, chopped

1 plum tomato, diced

½ green bell pepper, diced

1 tablespoon chopped jalapeño
    pepper (optional)

8 large eggs, lightly beaten

2 ounces Monterey Jack cheese,
    grated (about ½ cup)

2 ounces sharp Cheddar cheese,
    grated (about ½ cup)

1 tablespoon minced fresh cilantro

Fresh salsa (see recipe, page 53), or
    store-bought salsa

There are two kinds of people in this world: those who eat sweet things for breakfast and those who prefer savories. If you're the latter, this traditional Texas border recipe is for you (it has salty, crispy tortilla chips mixed right in!). Cookbook contributor Salma Abdelnour developed it based on the diner migas she ate as a child near the tumbleweedy west Texas town where the James Dean classic *Giant* was filmed. Making these on a Sunday morning still puts her in the mood for a Western epic or two.

1. In a large skillet, heat oil over moderate heat. Put in one tortilla strip to test the heat level; the oil is ready when the tortilla starts to sizzle as soon as you drop it in. Put the remaining tortilla strips in the pan and cook, stirring constantly, until they're crisp and slightly browned, about 3 minutes. Using a slotted spoon, remove them from the skillet and lay them on a plate lined with paper towels. Sprinkle with ½ teaspoon of salt.

2. Discard all but about 2 tablespoons oil from the skillet. Add the onion, tomato, pepper, and jalapeño, if using, and cook, stirring a few times, until softened, about 6 minutes. Add the eggs and stir, then add the tortilla strips and cook, stirring often, for around 4 minutes, until lightly scrambled, being careful not to overcook the eggs.

3. Stir in cheeses and cook until melted, about 1 minute. Remove pan from heat. Sprinkle with the cilantro and remaining ½ teaspoon salt and serve with salsa on the side.

Wake Up and Make Up Sausage Biscuits

Buttery Sausage Biscuits with Maple Syrup

You slept on it and you realize you were wrong. Or maybe not *wrong*, per se, but not entirely right. So let this generous home-made breakfast—a classic that was first published in *Glamour's Gourmet on the Run* in 1987—do the talking. Biscuits flecked with sausage and drizzled with maple syrup and butter will melt away any grudges.

Makes 6 biscuits

¼ pound sweet Italian sausage
1 cup all-purpose flour
1½ teaspoons baking powder
¼ teaspoon baking soda
¼ teaspoon salt
⅛ teaspoon freshly ground black pepper
2 tablespoons cold butter, diced into ¼-inch cubes, plus extra for serving
¼ cup buttermilk
Maple syrup, for serving

1. Preheat the oven to 450°F. Remove the sausage from its casing. Crumble the meat into a small heavy skillet, and cook over medium-high heat, stirring to break up any lumps, until it loses its pink color, about 8 to 10 minutes. Let cool slightly.

2. In a small bowl, combine the flour, baking powder, baking soda, salt, and pepper. Using your fingers, rub the diced cold butter into the flour mixture to form coarse crumbs.

3. Scrape the sausage and any pan drippings into the flour mixture. Pour in the buttermilk and stir just until the dough begins to form, then stop mixing to avoid overworking the dough.

4. Dust your palms with flour. On a well-floured surface, knead the dough 2 or 3 times until smooth, then pat or roll out to a ¾-inch thickness.

[CONTINUED]

5. Using a 2½-inch biscuit cutter or water glass, cut out 6 biscuit rounds. If any scraps remain, gather them up and pat them out again to a ¾-inch thickness, and cut out more rounds. Place the rounds on ungreased cookie sheets. Bake 9 to 12 minutes. While still warm, cut the biscuits open horizontally, and add a pat of butter and a drizzle of maple syrup. Serve.

6. To reheat the biscuits the next day, wrap loosely in aluminum foil, then warm in a 250°F oven for 10 to 15 minutes.

glamour girl tip

Instead of drizzling the cut biscuits with maple syrup, you can also make breakfast sandwiches by adding a slice of cheese and a fried egg (see Big Day Steak and Eggs, page 26, for the how-to on perfect frying).

Impress a Crowd Home Fries

Spicy Indian-Style Potatoes

These bright yellow, fiery-hot home fries are the Christian Louboutin heels of breakfast food: colorful, rich, and delicious to look at as well as to eat. The jalapeño, cayenne, and curry combine to create a fantastic heat. And while they do make a great A.M. side dish alongside eggs, they're sophisticated enough to serve with steak or chicken in the P.M. too.

1. In a large saucepan, cover the potatoes with cold water and add a large pinch of salt. Bring to a boil and let cook for 1 minute. Drain.

2. In large skillet, heat 1 tablespoon olive oil over moderate heat. Add the garlic and onions and cook until pale golden, stirring a few times, about 4 minutes.

3. Add the potatoes and jalapeño to the skillet along with another tablespoon of olive oil, $\frac{1}{2}$ teaspoon salt, and $\frac{1}{2}$ teaspoon black pepper. Turn up the heat to moderately high. As many of the potatoes as possible should be touching the bottom of the pan. Cook for 4 minutes without stirring.

4. Add the turmeric, cayenne, and curry powder to the skillet, and stir until the potatoes are well coated with the spices

Serves 2 as an entrée or 4 as a side dish

1 pound Yukon Gold or russet potatoes, scrubbed and cut into ½-inch cubes

Salt

4 tablespoons olive oil

2 garlic cloves, finely chopped

2 small red or yellow onions, chopped

1 small or ¼ large jalapeño pepper, seeded and minced (about 1 teaspoon)

Freshly ground black pepper

½ teaspoon turmeric

½ teaspoon cayenne

½ teaspoon curry powder

2 tablespoons minced flat-leaf parsley (optional)

[CONTINUED]

and turn bright yellow. Drizzle 1 tablespoon olive oil over the potatoes and let cook, without stirring, another 4 minutes.

5. By now, a crust should be starting to form on the edges of the potatoes. Stir to expose more potatoes to the bottom of the skillet so they continue to form a crust, and cook for about 5 minutes longer.

6. Remove from the heat, stir in the remaining tablespoon of olive oil, and season with salt and black pepper to taste. Sprinkle the parsley on top (if using).

It's Cocktail Hour *Somewhere*
Bourbon French Toast

Brioche French Toast with Maple-Bourbon Syrup

You may think booze before noon sounds strange (actually, we hope you do), but a splash of bourbon gives this French toast recipe its wonderfully earthy sweetness. It was first published in *Glamour's Gourmet on the Run*, and we've been treating ourselves to it on weekend mornings ever since.

1. In a shallow bowl or pie plate, whisk the eggs, milk, bourbon, orange zest, flour, cinnamon, and nutmeg until thoroughly combined.

2. In a large griddle or skillet, melt the butter over moderate heat, tilting to coat the griddle.

3. Dip the bread, one slice at a time, into the egg mixture, turning to coat both sides and giving each side a few seconds to soak. Transfer the slices to the griddle.

4. Cook the bread over moderate heat, until golden and slightly crisp, about 2 or 3 minutes on each side. Add more butter as needed to prevent the bread from sticking.

[CONTINUED]

Serves 2

FRENCH TOAST

3 large eggs

½ cup milk

1 tablespoon bourbon

Grated zest of 1 orange (see Glamour Girl Tip on page 34 for how to zest) or 1 teaspoon orange juice

½ cup all-purpose flour

⅛ teaspoon ground cinnamon

Pinch of ground nutmeg

1 teaspoon butter

Four 1-inch-thick slices brioche, challah, French bread, or white bread

Sliced strawberries (optional)

A few fresh mint leaves (optional)

BOURBON SYRUP

⅓ cup maple syrup

1 tablespoon bourbon

1 tablespoon butter

5. Meanwhile, make the bourbon syrup: In a small saucepan, combine the maple syrup, bourbon, and butter. Cook over moderately low heat until the butter is melted, about 3 minutes.

6. Arrange the French toast on plates. Pour the syrup over, garnish with strawberries and mint leaves (if using), and serve.

glamour girl tip

To make orange zest, just rub the medium-fine side of a grater over the orange skin, stopping when you get to the white stuff (called the pith).

Love You Pancakes

Classic Pancakes with Butter and Maple Syrup

Caroline Campion is the culinary superhero of the *Glamour* staff. By day, she's the books editor. By night, she is the pen (and pans) behind one of our favorite food blogs, devilandegg.com. Caroline believes pancakes are little declarations of affection and makes these (she doubles the recipe) for her husband and two children almost every weekend.

Serves 2

2 cups all-purpose flour

¼ teaspoon salt

1 tablespoon granulated sugar

1 tablespoon baking powder
   (or ½ teaspoon baking soda if
   you're going to use buttermilk)

2 large eggs

2 cups milk (or buttermilk)

1 to 2 tablespoons unsalted butter,
   plus more for serving

Confectioners' sugar, for dusting

Maple syrup and/or jam, for serving

1. In a medium bowl, mix together the flour, salt, granulated sugar, and baking powder. In a separate bowl, beat the eggs with 1½ cups of the milk (or see the Glamour Girl Tip on page 37 for instructions on how to make the pancakes even fluffier by separating the whites and yolks). Add the milk mixture to the flour mixture and mix just until combined. Don't overmix or the pancakes will be tough—blend just enough to get the flour moist, even if the mixture stays a bit lumpy. You can add up to ½ cup more regular milk (not buttermilk) to thin the batter if necessary.

2. Let the batter sit for 10 minutes to settle.

3. Heat a large nonstick skillet or lightly oiled cast-iron skillet over moderately low heat. Melt ½ tablespoon butter at the center of the skillet where you will spoon the batter (optional).

[CONTINUED]

4. Spoon about ¼ cup batter into the hot skillet directly onto the melted butter; your pancake should be about the size of a hockey puck.

5. Cook the pancake until the bottom is golden brown and the bubbles on the surface begin to break, about 2 minutes. Using a spatula, flip the pancake quickly. ("Have the courage of your convictions!" as Julia Child used to say.) Cook until golden brown, about 1 minute longer.

6. Transfer the finished pancake to a plate, cover with foil, and keep warm on the stove while you cook the rest of the batter. Add additional finished pancakes to the plate, cover, and keep warm.

7. Serve the pancakes dusted with confectioners' sugar. Pass butter, syrup, and/or jam at the table.

VARIATION: RASPBERRY-RICOTTA PANCAKES

1 lemon
1 pint fresh or frozen
  raspberries (thawed)
⅓ cup plus 1 tablespoon sugar
2 cups all-purpose flour
¼ teaspoon salt
1 tablespoon baking powder
1 cup part-skim ricotta cheese
1¼ cups milk
4 large eggs
Maple syrup, for serving

Caroline's raspberry-ricotta pancakes, a variation on the classic recipe above, are lighter and more sophisticated. But while the pancakes look bed-and-breakfast special, you can get all the ingredients in your local grocery store (frozen raspberries work if fresh are not in season).

1. Working over a medium bowl, using a box grater or a microplane, grate the zest from the lemon, being careful not to remove any of the bitter white pith. Cut the zested lemon into wedges and set them aside.

2. Add the raspberries to the bowl with the lemon zest. Stir in ⅓ cup sugar, gently crushing the raspberries with a

wooden spoon. Set aside to macerate while making the batter.

3. In a medium bowl, combine the flour, salt, 1 tablespoon sugar, and baking powder. In another bowl, beat the ricotta with the milk and eggs (or see the Glamour Girl Tip below for instructions on how to make the pancakes fluffier by separating the whites and yolks). Add the ricotta mixture to the flour mixture and stir until just combined. Let the batter sit for 10 minutes. Gently fold in the raspberries with their juices.

4. To cook the pancakes, follow steps 3 through 5 for the classic pancakes recipe on page 35.

5. Serve the finished pancakes with maple syrup and lemon wedges.

glamour girl tip

Caroline's Belgian grandma, Mamy, was a brilliant home cook who made everything from sorbet to rabbit stew in her tiny Brussels apartment. She taught Caroline the following make-'em-fluffy trick for *any* kind of pancake: Separate the whites and the yolks of the eggs and add just the yolks when the recipe calls for the eggs. Then beat the whites until stiff peaks form. Gently fold them into the batter at the end, once all other ingredients are combined.

I'm So Healthy Smoothie

Honeydew, Pineapple, and Mint Smoothie

Serves 2

2½ cups chopped fresh honeydew
   melon
1 cup chopped fresh or canned
   pineapple, drained
1 tablespoon agave syrup or honey
1 tablespoon chopped fresh mint
⅓ cup ginger ale, lemon-lime soda,
   club soda, soy milk, or yogurt
Salt
6 ice cubes

Smoothies have gotten a bad rap lately—not surprising, since many commercially made ones have more calories than a cheeseburger. But when you make them at home, *you're* in charge, and few things are as refreshing as freshly blended fruit. We've added ginger ale to give ours a little fizz, but if you want an even lower-cal version, use club soda, or even soy milk or yogurt.

In a blender, combine the fruit, agave syrup, mint, ginger ale, a pinch of salt, and the ice cubes. Blend until smooth and frothy. Pour into tall glasses and serve.

Invite Me Back Muffins

Moist Blueberry Muffins with Crunchy-Sweet Crumble

So you've finally finagled the invitation to your boss's weekend place or your poshest friends' lake retreat. Good Guest 101: Nothing says "I'm so glad to be here" like a batch of these muffins. The recipe calls for so many berries, every bite will be packed with burst-in-your-mouth goodness. And the streusel-like crumble on top just begs to be eaten all on its own. The muffins stay fresh for days—if they're not devoured as soon as you arrive.

1. Preheat the oven to 450°F. Spray a 12-cup muffin tin with cooking spray or line the cups with paper or foil liners; you can also use eight 5-ounce ramekins, spritzed with cooking spray, instead.

2. Make the crumble topping (if using): In a medium bowl, using your fingers, mix all of the crumble ingredients until small clumps form. Put the mixture in the freezer to chill and firm up while you work on the batter.

3. Make the muffins: In a medium bowl, combine the flour, baking powder, and salt. In a large bowl, with a mixer on high speed, beat the butter and sugar until creamy. Add the eggs one at a time and beat on medium speed between additions until smooth. Add the flour mixture in 2 batches,

Makes 12 medium or
8 jumbo muffins

CRUMBLE TOPPING (OPTIONAL)

½ cup sugar

⅓ cup all-purpose flour

1½ teaspoons ground cinnamon

¼ cup butter, melted

MUFFINS

2 cups all-purpose flour

2 teaspoons baking powder

½ teaspoon salt

1 stick unsalted butter (½ cup), softened

1 cup sugar

2 eggs

⅔ cup milk

2 cups fresh or frozen blueberries (if using frozen, do not defrost them first, but toss them in a few teaspoons of flour before stirring them into the mix in step 3)

alternating with the milk, beating on low speed between additions until just combined. Fold in the blueberries.

4. Spoon the batter into the prepared cups, filling all the way to the top. Sprinkle with the crumble topping (if using). Bake for 5 minutes. Reduce the oven temperature to 375°F and bake for about 20 minutes longer, until the muffins spring back when lightly touched with a finger. Set the pan on a rack and let cool for 15 minutes. Carefully remove the muffins from the pan, running the flat side of a knife gently around their sides to loosen them, if necessary.

glamour girl tip

The muffin batter can also be mixed by hand; just be sure the butter is truly soft, and blend the ingredients thoroughly.

Bring It Anywhere Banana Bread

Homestyle Banana Bread with Applesauce and Cinnamon

Glamour photo assistant Joanna Muenz, who also writes the charming food blog simplysifted.com, has been making banana bread since elementary school. She loves that it's a culinary multitasker—perfect for breakfast, nice for snack time, and delish for dessert, with a dollop of whipped cream. This version calls for applesauce instead of butter and only the whites of the eggs, so it has all of the luscious moistness without the extra calories.

Serves 4 to 6

3 ripe bananas
½ cup applesauce
4 egg whites
1 teaspoon vanilla extract
½ cup granulated sugar
½ cup light brown sugar
2 cups all-purpose flour
1 tablespoon ground cinnamon
1 teaspoon baking soda
¾ teaspoon baking powder
¼ cup vegetable oil

1. Preheat the oven to 350°F. Lightly grease a 9- by 5-inch loaf pan. Using a blender or an electric mixer, mash the bananas. Add the applesauce, egg whites, vanilla, and both sugars. Blend until smooth.

2. In a medium bowl, mix the flour, cinnamon, baking soda, and baking powder. Slowly add the banana mixture to the flour mixture and stir until just combined, then stir in the oil gently, until just blended.

3. Pour the batter into the prepared loaf pan, and bake for 50 to 55 minutes. Test for doneness with a toothpick. Cool for 15 minutes before serving.

glamour girl tip

Bananas get sweeter as they ripen. When Joanna finds the coveted mushy, spotty ones, she peels them, tosses them in a Ziploc bag, and freezes them for up to 6 months, to use in future cooking sessions.

kitchen basics:

Five Breakfasts for Very Busy Women

No time for an omelet or French toast? Some of our favorite morning meals take only seconds.

SAVORY AVOCADO SANDWICH

1 slice multigrain bread
½ avocado, sliced
Olive oil
Sea salt
Dried red pepper flakes

1. Toast bread and top with avocado, olive oil, and a pinch each of sea salt and red pepper flakes. The combo will give you energy and keep your mid-morning cravings in check.

MIDDLE EASTERN DELIGHT

1 quart plain low-fat yogurt
1 to 2 pieces of pita bread
Olive oil
Sea salt
Dried mint or oregano

1. The night before, set a colander lined with cheesecloth over a bowl, and pour in the quart of yogurt. Refrigerate overnight. The next morning, your colander will be filled with a mound of creamy, thick Middle Eastern spread called labneh.

2. Spread a spoonful of labneh on pita bread. Sprinkle it with a few drops of olive oil, a pinch of sea salt, and some dried mint or oregano if you like.

WINTER WARMER

This hearty oatmeal is easy, has a wonderfully nutty texture, and will keep you going all morning. You can make it super-fast, even without buying those just-add-water instant oatmeal packets.

1. Mix oats with brown sugar, cinnamon, and a dash of salt.

2. If using regular oats, add water and microwave for three minutes; for quick-cooking oats add boiling water and just stir it in. Let the oatmeal rest for a minute or two, then drizzle it with a bit of honey and fresh or dried fruit and nuts.

½ cup oats (either regular or quick-cooking)
1 tablespoon brown sugar
¼ teaspoon ground cinnamon
Salt
½ to ¾ cup water (depending on how thick you like your oatmeal)
Honey
Fresh or dried fruit
Nuts

INSTANT ENERGY FRUIT CUP

1. Cut apple and pear into bite-size chunks and place in a bowl. Add grapes, along with honey and lemon juice. Throw in sliced kiwi or pomegranate seeds if you have them.

2. Toss, and voilà: a 5-minute fruit cup, loaded with juiciness and fiber.

½ apple
½ pear
½ cup red seedless grapes
1 tablespoon honey
½ tablespoon fresh lemon juice
Sliced kiwi
Pomegranate seeds

MAD DASH PB&A

1. If you have exactly ten seconds to get out the door, chop an apple in half, then smear on some peanut butter. The pairing of fiber-rich carbohydrates from the apple and protein from the peanut butter takes longer to digest than just carbs alone, so you'll feel the energy lift for longer.

Spoonful of peanut butter
1 apple

nibbles

Any Excuse for a Party
Pigs in a Blanket

Cocktail Sausages with Rosemary and Spicy Mustard

Can anyone really resist pork wrapped in pastry? Fine. Good for them. *We* can't. Try this twist, which uses mini sausages that you sauté with fresh rosemary and serve with spicy Dijon mustard for dipping. The updated version is grown-up enough to impress your most sophisticated friends, but close enough to the original to leave your inner child (or *any* child) satisfied.

Serves 8 to 10

2 tablespoons olive oil

18 to 20 cocktail sausages, such as Vienna sausages (breakfast sausages cut into 2-inch lengths are fine too, as are full-size smoked sausages cut thickly on the bias into 2-inch lengths)

1 teaspoon minced fresh rosemary

Cooking spray

2 packages prepared crescent roll dough

Dijon mustard, for serving

1. Preheat the oven to 375°F.

2. Heat the olive oil in a cast-iron skillet over moderately high heat. Add the sausages and cook, stirring a few times, until browned on all sides, about 5 minutes; if using uncooked sausage, cook for another 10 to 12 minutes. In the last 2 minutes, stir in the rosemary. Transfer the sausages to a plate lined with paper towels and set aside.

3. Lightly coat a baking sheet with cooking spray. Unroll the crescent rolls and cut each triangle into 3 equal strips. Set the sausages on the strips and roll up. Arrange the sausage rolls 2 inches apart on the prepared baking sheet.

4. Bake for about 15 minutes, rotating the baking sheet halfway through, until the dough is puffed up and golden brown. Serve immediately, with Dijon mustard on the side. Refrigerate any leftover crescent dough for breakfast.

Hostess-in-a-Hurry Crostini

Broiled Baguette Toasts with Assorted Toppings

Serves 8

2 large baguettes, sliced into ¾-inch
thick pieces
4 garlic cloves, peeled and cut in half
crosswise
Olive oil for drizzling
Kosher salt and freshly ground black
pepper

Former *Glamour* editor and cookbook contributor Erin Zammett Ruddy loves to entertain, but always manages to underestimate how long it takes to get the meal on the table. She rarely serves dinner before 9:00 P.M. (or, if she's being completely honest, even later). That said, her guests never starve, thanks to her signature starters: little toasts (aka crostinis) with yummy things piled on top. You can literally put anything on these cuties—even the white bean dip from page 54—to make an instant hors d'oeuvre that will keep your guests happy till dinner. Whenever that is!

1. Preheat the broiler.

2. Working in batches, arrange the baguette slices on a baking sheet (you can line the sheet with foil for easier cleanup).

3. Place the baking sheet under the broiler for 1½ to 2 minutes, until the baguette slices are just golden. Remove the baking sheet from the broiler, and using tongs, flip the slices. Return the baking sheet to the broiler and toast for 1 minute longer. Watch closely so the toasts don't burn.

4. Pierce a garlic clove half with a fork so that the cut side is facing outward. Use the cut side to rub the toasts. (If the toasts are too hot to handle, hold them with a kitchen towel). Replace the garlic clove with a fresh half as needed.

5. Drizzle the toasts with olive oil and sprinkle with a little salt and pepper. Then add one of the toppings below or your own favorite combination. (The toppings below are well seasoned, so you may not need to salt and pepper the bread before you add them.)

TOPPINGS

TOMATO AND BASIL CROSTINI

In a medium bowl, mix together tomatoes, basil, capers, and red onion. Drizzle with olive oil and add kosher salt and freshly ground pepper to taste. Spoon onto toasts.

2 medium tomatoes, diced
1½ tablespoons chopped basil leaves
1 tablespoon roughly chopped capers
½ tablespoon finely chopped red onion

PARMIGIANO-REGGIANO, ARTICHOKE, AND LEMON-MAYO CROSTINI

Pile 1 teaspoon Parmigiano-Reggiano on each toast and broil it until melted, about 1 minute. Top each toast with a quartered artichoke heart, and drizzle with a bit of lemon-mayonnaise sauce (1 tablespoon mayonnaise blended with 1 tablespoon lemon juice, and a pinch each of kosher salt and freshly ground black pepper).

8 teaspoons freshly grated
   Parmigiano-Reggiano cheese
2 artichoke hearts from a jar, drained
   and quartered
1 tablespoon mayonnaise
1 tablespoon lemon juice

LEMONY GOAT CHEESE WITH OLIVES AND DILL CROSTINI

Mix 4 ounces goat cheese with 1 to 1½ teaspoons lemon zest and a pinch of freshly ground black pepper. Spread onto toasts and top each with 1 teaspoon chopped kalamata olives and a few sprigs of fresh dill.

4 ounces goat cheese, at room
   temperature
1½ teaspoons lemon zest
8 teaspoons chopped kalamata olives
Fresh dill

[CONTINUED]

OTHER TOPPING VARIATIONS

Try goat cheese topped with sliced, roasted red peppers from a jar or cream cheese topped with smoked salmon and dill.

glamour girl tip

To make lemon zest, just rub the medium-fine side of a grater over the lemon skin, stopping when you get to the white stuff (called the pith).

Super Bowl Guacamole

Tangy Avocado Dip with Red Onion, Cilantro, and Lime

This crowd-pleasing guac can be made ahead of time so you don't miss a minute of the game (or the commercials, if that's your thing!). To keep it from turning brown before you eat it, cover the guac with plastic wrap, making sure the plastic touches the surface, until you're ready to serve it.

Serves 4

2 ripe avocados, halved and pitted

1 tablespoon fresh lime juice

¼ cup finely chopped red or Vidalia onion

¼ cup chopped fresh cilantro

1 jalapeño pepper, seeded and finely chopped (optional)

½ cup finely chopped tomato (optional)

Salt

Tortilla chips, for serving

1. Scoop the avocados from their shells into a serving bowl. Sprinkle them with lime juice. Using a potato masher or a fork, mash them to a coarse puree.

2. Stir in the onion and cilantro, along with the jalapeño and tomato (if using); add salt to taste and additional lime juice, if desired. Serve with tortilla chips.

glamour girl tip

To judge the ripeness of an avocado, just give it a squeeze: the flesh should give a little when you press on it but not be too soft.

Make It in the Car Artichoke Dip

Creamy Artichoke and Cheese Party Dip

Serves 4

One 6-ounce jar marinated artichoke
   hearts
½ cup freshly grated Parmigiano-
   Reggiano cheese
¼ cup mayonnaise (no Miracle Whip!)
¼ cup sour cream
1 tablespoon minced flat-leaf parsley,
   plus more for garnish (optional)
Salt and freshly ground black pepper
Crackers or baguette slices, for
   serving

Glamour.com editor Lindsey Unterberger invented this moveable mini feast one evening while running late to a friend's birthday celebration. She does the stirring part of the recipe in the car (she's not the one driving!), and then microwaves it when she gets to the party. All her friends love it; yours will, too.

1. At home, drain the artichoke hearts and coarsely chop them.

2. Transfer to a medium bowl and add the Parmigiano-Reggiano, mayonnaise, sour cream, and parsley. (Now's the moment you can head to the car if you need to.) Mix until combined. If preparing this more than a half hour before you leave for the party, refrigerate until ready to use. Salt and pepper to taste.

3. Once you're near a microwave, cook on high for 1 minute and 30 seconds until the cheese has melted, stirring at 30-second intervals to ensure even heating. (Since microwave cooking times vary, you may need an additional 20 or 30 seconds to melt the cheese adequately.) Garnish with additional minced parsley and black pepper, if desired. Serve with crackers or a sliced baguette.

Yes, I Make My Own Salsa

Fresh Homemade Salsa with Tomato, Cilantro, and Jalapeño

Much as we love the ease of store-bought salsa, it pales in comparison to the DIY kind. Literally. The bright colors of these fresh ingredients amp up the look as well as the flavor. All you need are four ingredients and a sharp knife—or a box grater. When *Glamour* senior beauty editor Baze Mpinja made this salsa for her Cinco de Mayo party, she had to refill the bowl four times to keep up with her guests' insatiable scooping. Be warned!

Makes about 3 cups

4 large plum tomatoes, halved
½ small red onion
¼ cup chopped fresh cilantro
¼ jalapeño pepper, minced (or less, to taste), or hot sauce, to taste
Salt and freshly ground black pepper
Fresh lime juice

1. Remove the pulp and seeds from the tomatoes (by gently squeezing the halves), then cut them into ½-inch cubes; alternatively, for a less chunky salsa, grate them on the large holes of a box grater, discarding any leftover skins. You can use a food processor instead, but make sure not to overly puree the tomatoes.

2. Cut the onion into ¼-inch dice or grate on the large holes of a box grater.

3. In a serving bowl, combine the tomatoes and onion with the cilantro and jalapeño (or hot sauce to taste). Mix well, and add salt, pepper, and lime juice to taste.

Get Skinny Dip

Lemony White Bean Dip with Arugula, Garlic, and Sea Salt

Serves 4 to 6

3 cups packed arugula

3 to 4 garlic cloves

2 to 3 tablespoons olive oil

2 tablespoons lemon juice

Salt and freshly ground black pepper

One 15-ounce can white beans, such as cannellini or Great Northern beans, preferably low-sodium

Whole wheat crackers, pita chips, or toasted pita bread, for serving

As *Glamour's* health blogger, Sarah Jio is always searching for new snacks that A) are healthy, but B) don't taste like cardboard. This recipe is a winner on both counts. The arugula provides plenty of peppery flavor and the white beans are packed with fiber—which keeps you fuller longer. The dip in fact is so rich, you will not be able to tell it's good for you. No one will.

1. In a food processor, combine the arugula, garlic cloves, olive oil, and lemon juice with ¼ teaspoon salt and pulse until smooth.

2. Add the beans and pulse until they are chunky, not pureed. Scrape into a serving bowl and season with salt and pepper to taste. Serve with whole wheat crackers, pita chips, or toasted pita bread.

glamour girl tip

This dip can also be made in a blender. Just chop the arugula before pureeing it, for a smoother consistency.

Dinner's Coming Glazed Nuts

Nuts Spiked with Cinnamon and Cayenne

Cookbook contributor Salma Abdelnour spent years as an editor at *Food & Wine* magazine and writes a blog called SalmaLand, where she tells people where to eat out in New York. She's got serious foodie cred, so when she invites friends over for dinner, they come—hungry. While she's whipping up something fantastic, like Moroccan couscous with lamb (page 114), she puts out this bowl of nuts. A little bit spicy, a little bit sweet, they are the perfect way to stave off hunger. Make 'em yourself—and watch 'em disappear.

Makes 2½ cups

3 tablespoons sugar
½ teaspoon ground cinnamon
½ teaspoon cayenne
¼ teaspoon ground nutmeg
½ teaspoon salt
2 tablespoons butter
2½ cups nuts, such as almonds, pecans, walnuts, hazelnuts, and/or cashews (or a mix), shelled

1. In a small bowl, mix the sugar, spices, and salt.

2. Line a large rimmed baking sheet with wax paper. In a large skillet, heat the butter over moderate heat until melted. Add the nuts and cook, stirring, until darkened and fragrant, about 5 minutes. If the nuts begin to darken too quickly, lower the heat.

3. Add the spice mixture to the nuts, and cook over low heat, stirring frequently, until richly fragrant and toasted, about 10 minutes longer. You've got to watch the pan constantly since you'll be heating sugar, which burns quickly.

4. Spread the nuts out onto the prepared baking sheet and let cool. Break up the nuts before serving.

Two-Bite Tea Sammies

British-Style Crustless Tea Sandwiches

Makes 16 tea sandwiches

SANDWICHES

8 thin slices white sandwich bread,
   crusts removed

SPREAD

3 ounces cream cheese

2 tablespoons chopped chives or dill

1 teaspoon lemon juice

Salt and freshly ground pepper

CUCUMBER AND SALMON TOPPING

1 thinly sliced seedless cucumber

¼ pound thinly sliced smoked salmon

PROSCIUTTO TOPPING

¼ pound thinly sliced prosciutto

**CUCUMBER AND WATERCRESS
   TOPPING**

1 thinly sliced seedless cucumber

Watercress leaves

There are many things that *Glamour* editorial development director Susan Goodall, who is half-British, likes about tea sandwiches. They're tiny, tidy, and require no more than two bites, she says—making them the perfect midafternoon snack. A proper tea sandwich, she adds, is also never overstuffed with filling, meaning no drips, stains, or mess if you're serving to guests. But you know what's best about these mini meals? "They're cute," says Susan. "And there isn't enough cute food in this world."

1. Stir together ingredients for the spread mixture.

2. Spread 4 bread slices with about 1 tablespoon of cream cheese mixture. Top each slice with your choice of cucumber and salmon, prosciutto, or cucumber and watercress toppings.

3. Place the remaining 4 bread slices over the toppings and press together to form 4 sandwiches. Using a large serrated knife, cut each sandwich into 4 squares or triangles. Arrange tea sandwiches on a serving plate.

4. If you aren't serving the sandwiches right away, keep them moist by covering them with a damp paper towel and wrapping with a layer of plastic wrap. Keep chilled until ready to serve.

1. Combine all egg spread ingredients and spread on 4 bread slices instead of cream cheese mixture. Top each slice with prosciutto, watercress leaves, or smoked salmon (no cucumber). Place remaining 4 bread slices over the toppings and press together to form 4 sandwiches.

3 large hard-boiled eggs, shelled and finely chopped

1 teaspoon white truffle oil or a squirt of fresh lemon juice and sprinkling of chives or paprika

3 tablespoons mayonnaise

Salt and freshly ground pepper

glamour girl tip

Truffle oil is expensive. It'll run you between $10 and $25 for a small bottle at gourmet grocery stores or online from a vendor like amazon.com or Sur La Table. But should you buy it for this recipe, you may fall in love with its earthy, mushroomy flavor. Store it in the fridge; it should last three to six months. Besides using it in these tea sandwiches, you can add a teaspoon of truffle oil to mac and cheese or mashed potatoes. (Truffled mac and cheese is a current high-end restaurant obsession.) Bon appétit!

All-Grown-Up Deviled Eggs

Spice-Studded Deviled Eggs with Sweet Paprika

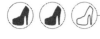

Serves 12

12 large eggs
½ cup mayonnaise
2 tablespoons finely chopped shallots
2 teaspoons red wine vinegar
2 teaspoons Dijon mustard
1 teaspoon Colman's mustard (dry)
1 tablespoon finely chopped chives
1 tablespoon finely chopped flat-leaf
  parsley
½ teaspoon curry powder
  (preferably Madras)
½ teaspoon salt
¼ teaspoon black pepper
⅛ teaspoon cayenne
Sweet smoked paprika, for sprinkling

When she's not crunching numbers as *Glamour*'s editorial business manager, Eilish Morley is a girl with a passion for vintage. "I'm really into the fifties," she says. "Furniture, dresses . . . I love anything with that retro-chic vibe, and these eggs definitely fit the bill." Eilish says serving deviled eggs at parties makes her feel like a grown-up—a grown-up who knows how to have a good time. For one thing, they're a little more sophisticated than chips and salsa. For another thing, the presentation looks fancy—but you can actually fake that swirly egg topping effect with a Ziploc bag.

1. In a large saucepan, combine the eggs with enough cold water to cover by 2 inches. Bring to a boil, then turn the heat down to low and cook the eggs for exactly 10 minutes. Carefully pour off the hot water, then shake the saucepan so the eggs bump into each other to crack the shells. Run cold water over the eggs until they are cool enough to handle.

2. Peel the eggs under running water. Cut the eggs in half lengthwise. Spoon out the egg yolks and add to a large bowl. Arrange the whites on a platter. Mash the yolks with a fork. Add the remaining ingredients except the paprika. Using a rubber spatula, stir the yolk mixture thoroughly until smooth and well blended.

3. Spoon the yolk mixture into a resealable plastic bag. Snip a ¼-inch triangle off the corner of the bag with scissors, then twist the bag to force the egg mixture toward the opening. Holding an egg white in one hand and the bag in the other, squeeze the egg yolk mixture into the halved egg white in a circular motion. Fill the remaining egg whites, then sprinkle with paprika. The eggs can be served immediately or covered and refrigerated up to 8 hours before serving.

kitchen basics:

How to Make a Perfect Cheese Plate

An artfully arranged cheese plate—to serve with drinks before dinner, or after, garnished with grapes—is a thing of beauty. It gives you a chance to show off your fabulous taste, even when you're running around at top speed trying to get dinner ready. Specialty cheese shops are magical places, but these days your local supermarket has decent choices too.

WHAT TO BUY

- Look for variety. Pick cheeses that are different in shape, size, color, and texture—ideally a mixture of firmer cheeses, like aged Gouda, manchego, or Parmigiano-Reggiano; and softer cheeses, like fresh mozzarella, taleggio, or chèvre (that's just French for goat cheese).

- Don't be shy. If you're not familiar with a cheese, ask for a taste of it at the shop before you commit to buying it. (At the supermarket, goat cheese, Parmigiano-Reggiano, and a blue cheese like Gorgonzola are smart bets.)

- Buy enough. Three kinds of cheese should be enough for a small get-together; for a larger gathering, pick up five or six varieties. As for quantity, count on each person eating 2 to 3 ounces of cheese total.

HOW TO ARRANGE IT

- Serve at room temperature. Cheeses simply taste best that way. At least an hour before the party, take the cheeses out of the fridge and keep them wrapped until serving time. Line them up on a platter or cutting board from mildest to strongest tasting, or just set them up in a way that pleases your eye.

- Give each cheese its own knife. You can cut a few slices of each cheese on the board, but leave the rest whole and let guests do the slicing.

WHAT TO SERVE ALONGSIDE

- Pair with crackers or bread. Walnut or raisin bread is fantastic, but other tricked-out breads and crackers that involve seeds or herbs will distract from the taste.

- Add extras: Try a bunch of red or golden grapes or sliced pears, toasted nuts, Medjool dates, or fresh figs. Chutneys like fig or mango, jams like tomato or sour cherry, and good-quality honey are delicious with cheese too. If you're serving the cheese plate as an hors d'oeuvre (not after dinner), savory extras like olives and roasted red peppers are nice go-withs, served in separate little bowls.

BUT REMEMBER . . .

You can add all these bells and whistles—or you can just buy three glorious cheeses and a baguette, and call it a day. Virtually everyone loves cheese, and everyone will be happy.

drinks

Breakfast in Bed Mimosa

Tropical Fruit Sorbet and Champagne Cocktail

If the last time you sipped a glass of anything in bed was when you were ten and had the flu, and the glass was filled with flat ginger ale and served to you by your mom, well—forget all that. For mornings that call for an adult breakfast in bed, whip this mimosa up in seconds. No, wait, better idea: Have someone *else* whip it up for you. *Glamour* staffer Ranya Barrett's husband, Dave, did just that on her birthday. "Heavenly," she reports. Good boy.

Serves 2

¼ cup passion fruit sorbet or mango sorbet, or more to taste
1 half-bottle chilled champagne or Prosecco

1. In the microwave or in a small saucepan, melt the sorbet over low heat, stirring occasionally, until just thawed. Pour 2 tablespoons sorbet into each of 2 champagne flutes.

2. Top the glasses with champagne or Prosecco, adding more sorbet, as desired, to sweeten the mimosa. Stir gently and serve right away.

Brunch at My Place Bloody Mary

Build Your Own Bloody Mary Bar, with Mix-ins and Garnishes

Serves 4

1½ cups tomato juice
¾ cup vodka
Juice of 1 lime (2 to 3 tablespoons)
2 tablespoons Worcestershire sauce
1 tablespoon prepared horseradish
⅛ teaspoon Tabasco
Salt to taste
Freshly ground pepper to taste
Ice cubes
Lime wedges, for garnish
Celery stalks, for garnish (optional)

Hieroglyphics suggest that Cleopatra sipped Bloody Marys while dishing with her best girlfriends, and medieval texts show King Arthur serving them when the Round Table was chillaxing. Neither of these things is true, of course—but they could be, since this drink's alchemy of vodka and tomato juice on the rocks has come to be code for relaxed, gab-filled meals. Bloody Marys are the perfect combination of savory, spicy, and tangy, and are one of those few drinks that really *can* be enjoyed in the morning.

1. In a large pitcher, combine all ingredients except ice and garnishes.

2. Fill glasses (preferably highball, but any tall glass will do) with ice, then pour in the Bloody Marys; garnish with lime wedges and/or celery stalks and serve.

glamour girl tip

If you're entertaining a group, set up a Bloody Mary bar and let your guests customize their own drinks instead of mixing them yourself. Place individual glasses on the bar next to a big bowl filled with ice. Present the tomato juice in a glass pitcher. Set a bottle of vodka next to it (or pour the vodka into a pitcher), and place a shot glass nearby so guests can measure their own quantity. Serve the Worcestershire, horseradish, Tabasco, salt, and pepper in small bowls with spoons, or line up all the ingredients in the containers they came in. Arrange the lime wedges and celery stalks in separate bowls.

Forget the Mistake You Made at Work Margarita

Pink Watermelon Margarita

"I'm sorry" works. So does "It'll never happen again." But for those nights when you're obsessing, we recommend . . . tequila. Mix up these babies and realize that you did not get fired. We all screw up sometimes. Kennedy had the Bay of Pigs; you had this. Feeling better? Drink more. Forgive self.

Serves 4

3 cups chopped watermelon
Juice of 10 limes (¾ to 1 cup)
⅓ cup sugar
2 cups ice cubes
1 cup tequila
½ cup Grand Marnier or triple sec

1. In a blender, combine the watermelon, lime juice, sugar, and ice and blend until smooth.

2. Add the tequila and Grand Marnier or triple sec and pulse to blend. (If your blender is too small, pour the blended watermelon mixture into a pitcher and stir in the alcohol.)

3. Fill tall glasses with more ice. Pour the margaritas over and serve.

glamour girl tip

To salt a glass, spread a thin layer of salt in a shallow dish. Moisten the edges of 4 glasses with a lime wedge and dip them in the salt. Tap the glasses to remove the excess salt, then fill them with ice and margarita mixture.

Man Trouble Mojito

White Rum and Mint Cocktail

Serves 2

20 mint leaves, plus 2 mint sprigs,
   for garnish
4 tablespoons fresh lime juice
   (from 2 to 3 limes), plus 2 lime
   slices, for garnish
2 tablespoons sugar
¼ cup white rum
Crushed ice
½ cup club soda

Three days after going out with a new guy she really liked, food blogger and photo assistant Joanna Muenz got this text: "Hey JoJo." Hmm. No one calls her JoJo. Was he being flirty? Or did he only see her as a friend? And why did he wait so long to send it, anyway? Joanna and her roommates debated—and made themselves a batch of these delicious rum cocktails along the way. In the end, they were still baffled, but at least they had a favorite new cocktail in common. Mix it up the next time ur txtd by a v confsng mn.

1. In each of two tall glasses, combine 8 to 10 mint leaves with 2 tablespoons fresh lime juice and 1 tablespoon sugar. Crush the mint leaves into the mixture with a wooden muddler or the back of a spoon until the sugar is fully dissolved.

2. Add ⅛ cup white rum to each glass, and lots of crushed ice. Top each glass with ¼ cup club soda and stir.

3. Garnish each glass with a mint sprig and a lime slice, and serve with a straw.

Glamour Gimlet

Cucumber Gimlet

Famed chef Charlie Palmer's bar and restaurant Aureole is twenty steps from *Glamour*'s office door. It's a luxe, and expensive, place, but the drinks are career-girl affordable. As a result, the bar has become our Cheers, and this cool cucumber cocktail is a staff favorite. Serve it at a cocktail party—ideally outdoors, in the summertime—and you'll feel miles and miles away from your in-box.

Serves 4

¼ cup plus 2 tablespoons sugar
¼ cup plus 2 tablespoons water
2 large cucumbers
1 cup gin
4 tablespoons fresh lime juice
    (from 2 to 3 limes)
1 cup ice cubes
4 lime slices

1. To make a simple syrup, combine the sugar and water in a small saucepan and bring to a boil, stirring until the sugar is fully dissolved. Remove from heat, transfer to a bowl, and refrigerate for 15 minutes, or until cool.

2. Meanwhile, slice four ¼-inch-thick slices from 1 cucumber, and set the slices aside. Peel and coarsely chop the remaining cucumber; puree the chopped pieces in a food processor until smooth. Place a fine strainer over a large bowl, and pour the puree into the strainer, pressing on the solids. Discard the solids.

3. Pour 1 cup of the resulting cucumber juice (you may have some left over) into a pitcher, along with the gin, lime juice, and chilled sugar syrup. Add the ice, and mix all the ingredients thoroughly.

[CONTINUED]

4. Strain into 4 small glasses (martini ones if you have them), and garnish each glass with lime slices and the reserved cucumber slices. (Optional: Dip the reserved cucumber slices in salt before using them as a garnish.) Serve.

glamour girl tip

If you don't want to make simple syrup, you can sweeten this cocktail with 3 tablespoons of agave. It may give the cocktail a slightly darker color, depending on the syrup you use.

Thanks for Helping Me Move Michelada

Spicy Mexican Beer Cocktail

If a Bloody Mary and a Corona had a baby, that baby would taste like a michelada. Spicy, salty, tangy, and thirst-quenching, this Mexican "beer cocktail" is the perfect thing to serve sweaty friends who've just helped you haul your overstuffed boxes. Pair it with some tostadas (p. 115) and homemade guac (page 51), and they'll probably help you unpack too!

If you're feeling lazy, you can make a simplified michelada just by mixing the lime juice and the beer—the result is refreshing, tasty, and *easy*.

Serves 2

Salt
⅓ cup fresh lime juice, plus 1 lime
 wedge
Ice cubes
Two 12-ounce bottles beer, preferably
 a Mexican beer like Corona
1½ teaspoons Worcestershire sauce
2 to 2½ teaspoons Tabasco or
 other favorite hot sauce
1 teaspoon soy sauce
Freshly ground pepper

1. Spread enough salt into a small, shallow plate so that it covers the bottom.

2. Run the lime wedge along the rims of two highball glasses or Mason jars to wet them, then dip the rims of the glasses into the salt.

3. Place a few ice cubes in each glass. Then, in each glass, pour a bottle of beer, half the lime juice, ¾ teaspoon Worcestershire, 1 teaspoon hot sauce (or slightly more if you like the drink extra-spicy), ½ teaspoon soy sauce, and salt and pepper to taste. Stir and serve.

xy City Cocktail

Classic Manhattan with Maraschino Cherries

Serves 2

Ice cubes

½ cup blended whiskey, such as
   Seagram's 7

¼ cup sweet vermouth

2 dashes angostura bitters

Maraschino cherries or 2 strips lemon
   zest, twisted, for garnish

Why is the Manhattan such a romantic classic? Let us count the reasons. There's the glamorous-sounding name ("I'll Take Manhattan!"). The lusciously grown-up taste (those bitters!). And the fact that both men and women seem to love the drink equally. Besides, it's *sexy*, a holdover from a world before Facebook flirting and friends with benefits... which is a world we all should visit every now and then.

1. Fill a cocktail shaker (or a tall glass) halfway with ice. Add all the ingredients except the garnish.

2. Shake (or stir well if you're mixing the drink in a glass) for 15 to 20 seconds, then strain into two martini glasses. Garnish each glass with a maraschino cherry or lemon twist and serve.

Style on a Budget White Sangría

Spanish Wine Cocktail with Fresh Fruit

It's one of the great freeing realizations of a woman's life: the understanding that *pricier* wines aren't always *better* wines. And it's true! You can get a great bottle of wine for under $15. We like sauvignon blanc from New Zealand, rioja from Spain, or syrah from California. Best of all, when your budget is especially tight, you can make delicious sangría out of cheap wine, and no one—but no one—will complain.

Serves 4

One 750-ml bottle dry white wine, such as sauvignon blanc or pinot grigio

½ to 1 cup brandy, to taste

¼ cup sugar

2 limes, sliced into thin rounds

2 lemons, sliced into thin rounds

1 orange, sliced into thin rounds

1 green apple, sliced

1 small bunch white grapes, removed from their stems, sliced in half

1 cup seltzer

Ice cubes

1. In a large glass pitcher, combine the wine, brandy, and sugar, stirring until the sugar is dissolved.

2. Add the fruit and seltzer to the pitcher. Let the sangría marinate in the refrigerator for 1 to 2 hours before serving. Add ice to the pitcher, stir, and serve.

Summer in a Glass Lemonade

Tart Nonalcoholic Strawberry Lemonade with Fresh, Sweet Berry Puree

Serves 6 to 8

⅔ cup sugar

5 cups cold water

Zest from 2 lemons

1 cup fresh lemon juice (from 5 to 7 lemons)

1 pint strawberries (fresh or frozen), chopped in half and with the hulls removed

2 dozen ice cubes

Our pregnant friends inspired this nonalcoholic drink. No matter how cute that baby bump gets, nine months without cocktails is a bummer. Enter this fruity twist on old-fashioned lemonade. It's *much* more special than seltzer—and, if anyone *is* drinking, also works nicely with a shot of rum mixed in.

1. In a medium saucepan, combine the sugar, 1 cup water, and the lemon zest. Simmer gently over moderate heat for 10 minutes; transfer to a bowl and let cool.

2. Strain the syrup into a 2-quart serving pitcher. Stir in the lemon juice and remaining 4 cups water.

3. In a blender, puree the strawberries.

4. Pour the strawberry puree into the pitcher, stir in the ice, and serve.

glamour girl tip

To make lemon zest, just rub the medium-fine side of a grater over the lemon skin, stopping when you get to the white stuff (called the pith).

soups & salads

Feel Better Fast Chicken Soup

Hot and Sour Chicken Soup with Cilantro and Snow Peas

Too sick to leave the couch? Get the man in your life to make this for you—the recipe is that easy. First published in *Glamour* in 2007, it has become a comfort-food favorite because it pairs that classic of grandmothers everywhere—chicken soup—with a modern, Asian-infused twist. The hot sauce will clear your head, and the leftovers are delicious enough to serve to guests . . . when you feel well enough to have them.

Serves 2 to 4

6 cups chicken stock or low-sodium broth
1 shallot, minced
2 garlic cloves, minced
1 teaspoon finely grated ginger
½ tablespoon Sriracha hot sauce (You can use *any* hot sauce, but we love this kind, available at most stores.)
1 bunch cilantro, rinsed and retied with string, plus ¼ cup minced fresh cilantro leaves for garnish (optional)
1 boneless, skinless chicken breast
3 tablespoons lime juice (from 1 to 2 limes)
½ cup Chinese snow peas or sugar snap peas, stems removed, peas chopped into 1-inch pieces
1 small bunch broccoli (optional), cut into florets
One 10-ounce box dried egg noodles (optional)
Salt and freshly ground pepper

1. In a medium casserole or Dutch oven, bring the chicken stock to a boil with the shallot, garlic, ginger, Sriracha, bunch of cilantro, and chicken breast. Turn the heat down to low and simmer for about 6 minutes.

2. Flip the breast over. Add the lime juice, snow peas, broccoli, and/or noodles (if using), and simmer until the chicken is cooked throughout, about 5 minutes, slightly longer for thicker chicken breasts. When the breast is fully cooked (slit it with a knife to make sure), use tongs to transfer to a cutting board and slice into thin, bite-size pieces.

3. Return the meat to the soup. Simmer for 5 minutes longer. Discard the bunch of cilantro and add salt, pepper, lime juice, and Sriracha to taste. Garnish with minced cilantro, if desired, and serve.

No Stove Required Gazpacho

Classic Tomato Gazpacho, with Sweet Corn and Mango Variations

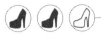

Serves 2 to 3

1 pound ripe tomatoes

1 cucumber, cut in half lengthwise, seeds scooped out

1 cup cold water

1 scallion, finely chopped

1 garlic clove, minced

¼ cup finely chopped fresh cilantro

2 tablespoons lime juice

1 tablespoon red wine vinegar or sherry vinegar

½ teaspoon salt

¼ teaspoon freshly ground black pepper

Plantain chips, for serving (optional)

Troy Dunham, who works in *Glamour's* art department, lives in a tiny apartment with no air-conditioning. Come summer, he used to put hazard tape on his oven and go into bunny mode: eating only salad, salad, and more salad. Until he learned to make gazpacho, that is. While classic gazpacho is red (made with tomatoes), we've added two fun yellow-orange variations here—a sweet corn gazpacho and a mango one as well. Troy serves them to friends with plantain chips, but they're also nice with a simple salad and baguette slices.

1. Roughly chop 1 tomato and 1 cucumber half, and puree them in a blender or food processor with the cold water. Pour the mixture through a wire-mesh sieve set over a large bowl, pressing on the solids. Discard the solids.

2. Finely chop the remaining tomatoes and cucumber half and add them to the bowl with the scallion, garlic, cilantro, lime juice, vinegar, salt, and pepper. Stir together, and chill until cold, about 1 hour. Serve with plantain chips, if desired.

VARIATION 1: SWEET CORN GAZPACHO

Instead of tomatoes, puree the kernels from 2 ears of corn (see the grilled shrimp recipe, page 138 for instructions on how to remove kernels from the cob) along with the chopped cucumber half and water. Pour the puree through a sieve into a bowl and stir in 1 cup corn kernels (from 1 or 2 ears of corn, depending on size), along with the remaining chopped cucumber half and 1 diced red bell pepper. Then stir in the remaining ingredients (scallion, garlic, cilantro, lime juice, vinegar, salt, and pepper) from the classic gazpacho recipe. Chill for an hour before serving.

3-4 ears corn (instead of tomatoes)
1 red bell pepper, diced

VARIATION 2: MANGO GAZPACHO

Instead of tomatoes, puree 1 peeled, pitted, and chopped ripe mango with the chopped cucumber half and water. Pour through a sieve into a bowl and stir in 1 additional peeled, pitted, and finely chopped mango along with the remaining chopped cucumber half. Instead of the scallion, stir in 3 tablespoons chopped red onion, then add the remaining ingredients (garlic, cilantro, lime juice, vinegar, salt, and pepper) from the classic gazpacho recipe. Chill for an hour before serving.

2 ripe mangos (instead of tomatoes)
3 tablespoons chopped red onion

glamour girl tip

Using local, farmstand tomatoes—or sweet cherry tomatoes—will take your gazpacho from good to great. If you can, chill the soup overnight to let the flavors deepen.

Welcome to My Villa Tuscan Bread Soup

Tomato Soup with Parmesan Cheese and Croutons

Serves 4

¼ cup olive oil

1 medium onion, finely chopped

4 garlic cloves , minced

One 28-ounce can whole tomatoes, drained and coarsely chopped, juice reserved

3 cups chicken stock or low-sodium broth

½ loaf Italian bread, cut into 1-inch cubes (3 cups)

1 cup water

1 tablespoon sugar

Salt and freshly ground pepper

⅓ cup thinly sliced fresh basil

¼ cup freshly grated Parmigiano-Reggiano cheese, for serving

There are certain easy, delicious dishes that are the building blocks of a confident home cook. You make them again and again, they turn out perfectly each time, and they give you the self-assurance to try new and more challenging dishes. This soup is just such a dish. You can serve it to friends and family, but it's also a wonderful meal to make for yourself: Pour it into a beautiful bowl and the bright red broth, sprinkled with basil and freshly grated Parmigiano-Reggiano cheese, gives you that great farm-to-table feeling, even though the main ingredient came out of a can.

1. In a medium saucepan, heat the oil over moderately high heat. Add the onion and garlic and cook, stirring, until softened, about 5 minutes. Stir in the tomatoes and reserved juice and simmer, stirring occasionally, for 15 minutes.

2. Add the stock, bread, water, sugar, ½ teaspoon salt, and ¼ teaspoon pepper to the saucepan and simmer, stirring occasionally, until the bread has absorbed the liquid and the soup is thick, about 20 minutes. If the soup feels too dense as it's cooking, add another cup of water. Stir in the basil, and add salt and pepper to taste. Ladle the soup into bowls, and top each bowl with about 1 tablespoon grated Parmigiano-Reggiano.

glamour girl tip

Supermarket Italian bread works just fine for this recipe.

Complexion Soup

Carrot Soup with Ginger and Lemongrass

Glamour's beauty editors call carrots "the friendliest skin food around." They've read the studies and they know: Carrots are packed with beta carotene, which repairs the skin, and loaded with vitamin C, an antioxidant that battles free radicals. This zingy, gingery soup is a delicious way to get your skin fix, and it's perfect with a salad for a light lunch.

1. In a large stockpot, heat the oil and butter over high heat. Add the garlic, onion, ginger, lemongrass (or lemon zest), coriander, cumin, and cinnamon. Cook for 5 minutes on medium heat, stirring constantly, until the onions soften, being careful not to let the mixture burn.

2. Increase the heat to moderately high. Add the carrots and 2 cups water to the stockpot and cook, covered, for about 15 minutes, stirring occasionally, until the vegetables are softened.

3. Add the stock to the stockpot and simmer for about 30 minutes.

4. Let the mixture cool for 5 minutes. Discard pieces of lemongrass. Working in two batches, ladle the soup into a blender or food processor and puree.

[CONTINUED]

Serves 2 to 3

2 tablespoons olive oil

1 tablespoon butter

2 garlic cloves, minced

1 large white onion, diced
   (about 1 cup)

3 tablespoons minced fresh ginger

2 fresh lemongrass stalks, chopped
   into one-inch pieces (or zest
   from 1 lemon)

1 tablespoon ground coriander

1 teaspoon ground cumin

1 teaspoon ground cinnamon

2½ pounds carrots, peeled and
   chopped

3½ cups water

4 cups vegetable stock

½ cup orange juice

½ cup light sour cream, plus
   2 to 3 teaspoons for garnish

Salt and freshly ground pepper,
   to taste

1 tablespoon minced chives,
   for garnish

5. Pour the pureed soup back into the stockpot. Add the orange juice, 1½ cups of water, and ½ cup sour cream to the stockpot. Stir until well blended. Add salt and pepper to taste.

6. Heat the mixture for 3 or 4 minutes over medium-low heat; you can also serve it cold. Ladle the soup into bowls, and garnish each with 1 teaspoon sour cream and a sprinkling of chives.

Baby, It's Cold Outside Crabmeat Soup

Tahitian-Style Crabmeat Soup with Coconut Milk

Most of the ingredients in this soup come from cans, but don't let that fool you. The end result is fresh, flavor-packed, and verrry upscale (one of our staffers snatched the recipe from a super-chic L.A. friend after eating it at her posh dinner party). Coconut milk, a common ingredient in tropical cuisines, gives the dish an island vacation flavor. Serve it with crusty bread or homemade croutons (see below) and get ready to write out the recipe for *your* guests.

Serves 4

1 medium onion, diced

4 tablespoons butter

One 13.5-ounce can coconut milk

1 cup heavy cream

1 cup chicken stock or low-sodium broth

1 pound lump crabmeat, picked free of shells

One 10-ounce package frozen chopped spinach

Salt and freshly ground pepper

Fresh lemon juice

1. In a large pot, cook the onion in the butter over moderately low heat until just softened, about 5 minutes. Reduce the heat to medium-low and add the coconut milk, cream, stock, crabmeat, and spinach.

2. Simmer for 30 minutes. Just before serving, add salt, pepper, and lemon juice to taste.

glamour girl tip

To add crunch, toss some homemade croutons into the soup. Dice a half baguette, small ciabatta, or Italian loaf, coat the pieces in plenty of olive oil, and put them on a rimmed baking sheet in a 400°F oven (or toaster oven) for 7 minutes, or until nicely browned and crunchy.

No More Takeout for You! Soup

Green Pea and Potato Soup with Sour Cream and Chives

Serves 8

2 medium leeks

2 tablespoons vegetable oil

2 large russet potatoes
(about 1 pound), peeled and cut
into 1-inch cubes

3 cups fresh or frozen peas

½ teaspoon sugar

4 cups vegetable broth

Salt and freshly ground pepper

1 small head iceberg lettuce, trimmed
and chopped (6 to 7 cups)

Lemon juice to taste (optional)

½ cup sour cream

Chopped fresh chives, for garnish

True story: During a particularly busy time in her life, cookbook editor Veronica Chambers had gotten into such a routine of ordering takeout that one night the delivery guy asked her out on a date. In an effort to be polite, she fudged and said, "Well, I have a boyfriend." To which he replied, "I'm here every night. You do *not* have a boyfriend." At that moment, she realized it was time to learn to cook, so she concocted this easy recipe. Make a big batch on Sunday, and you can heat up the leftovers in far less time than it takes to call for pizza.

1. Trim off and discard the roots and dark green tops of the leeks. Cut the leeks lengthwise in quarters, then crosswise into ½-inch pieces. Rinse thoroughly (see page 159 for a leek-cleaning tip).

2. In a large saucepan, heat the oil over moderate heat. Add the leeks and potatoes, and cook for 2 minutes, stirring. Add the peas, sugar, and broth. Bring the mixture to a boil over high heat, then reduce the heat to moderately low. Add salt and pepper to taste, then cover and simmer for 10 minutes.

3. Stir in the chopped lettuce. Cover and cook until the lettuce is wilted and the potatoes are tender, about 3 minutes. Working in batches, ladle the soup into a food processor and puree until smooth. Return the pureed soup to the saucepan

and stir over moderate heat. Add salt, pepper, and lemon juice to taste (if using).

4. Ladle the soup into serving bowls and top with a spoonful of sour cream and a sprinkling of chives.

glamour girl tip

When using any kind of store-bought broth, always look for the low-sodium versions. Most still have enough salt to be flavorful.

Ladies Who Lunch Salad

Mixed Greens with Roquefort Cheese, Pomegranate, and Rosemary-Lime Dressing

Serves 4

SALAD

6 cups mixed salad greens

¾ cup pomegranate seeds (from about 1 medium pomegranate)

1 Bosc pear, sliced lengthwise into ½-inch wedges and cored

½ cup crumbled Roquefort or other blue cheese

¼ cup chopped walnuts

DRESSING

3 tablespoons balsamic vinegar

Juice of 1 lime (about 2 to 3 tablespoons)

1 teaspoon sugar

2 teaspoons minced fresh rosemary, or 1 teaspoon dried

½ cup extra-virgin olive oil

Salt and freshly ground pepper

Glamour editors like to eat, but we also like to cook. After bonding at the office, in fact, two former staffers started a cooking club with four other women and wrote two cookbooks. This upscale salad recipe, which ran in the magazine in 2003, appears in one of them, *The Cooking Club Party Cookbook*. The mix is as pretty to look at as it is delicious to eat. It features regal ingredients (pomegranate seeds, rosemary, Roquefort), so even if you're not a *true* super-rich lady who lunches, you'll feel like one. Serve with a broiled baguette (page 48), and strawberry lemonade (page 74) or white sangría (page 73).

1. Make the salad: In a large bowl, combine all the salad ingredients.

2. Make the dressing: In a small bowl, whisk together the vinegar, lime juice, sugar, and rosemary. Slowly whisk in the olive oil until well mixed. Add salt and pepper to taste. Drizzle the dressing over the salad and serve. (You may have some dressing left over.)

glamour girl tip

You can buy pomegranate seeds in many stores, but harvesting the seeds from the actual fruit is easier than it looks. Cut the fruit into quarters, submerge under water in a bowl, and pick them out, then drain. No muss, no fuss!

No-Fail Kale Salad

Caesar-Style Salad with Kale, Pecorino Cheese, and Homemade Croutons

In an effort to bring readers the latest good-for-you foods, executive editor Wendy Naugle, who oversees our health coverage, is constantly sampling vitamin-rich, vegetable-laden fare. The only problem? She's more of a meat and potatoes kind of gal. Enter this salad. After tasting it at an event for health guru Andrew Weil's restaurant, True Food Kitchen, in Phoenix, Wendy fell in love. She calls it a sophisticated Caesar salad and the most painless way to eat lots of kale, which is good for you in a gazillion ways. Finally, something her health editor brain and her picky palate could agree on. Wendy has passed the recipe to friends, served it to dinner guests, and made it for herself dozens of times. And it always, always satisfies.

Serves 4

Juice of 1 lemon

6 tablespoons extra-virgin olive oil

2 garlic cloves, mashed

Salt and freshly ground black pepper

Red pepper flakes

4 to 6 loosely packed cups kale, preferably flat-leaf purple kale—midribs removed and leaves thinly sliced

⅔ cup grated Pecorino Toscano cheese (Rossellino variety if you can find it) or other flavorful grating cheese, such as Asiago or Parmigiano-Reggiano

1 small loaf ciabatta or other rustic bread, cut into 1-inch cubes (about 1 cup)

1. In a large serving bowl, whisk together the lemon juice, 4 tablespoons olive oil, garlic, salt and pepper to taste, and a generous pinch (or more, to taste) of red pepper flakes. Add the kale and toss well.

2. Add two-thirds of the cheese to the serving bowl and toss again. Let the salad rest for at least an hour. Yep, an hour—the dressing softens the sturdy kale to give it a more delicate romaine-like texture.

3. Preheat the oven to 400°F.

[CONTINUED]

4. Toss the bread in the remaining 2 tablespoons olive oil (or use garlic-infused olive oil, if you have it). Spread the bread cubes on a rimmed baking sheet. Toast in the oven for 7 minutes, until golden. Remove from the oven and cool on a plate lined with paper towels.

5. After the salad has rested, add the bread cubes, toss the salad again, top with the remaining cheese, and serve.

It's All About the Dressing Salad

Arugula and Grapefruit Salad with Shallot Vinaigrette

When cookbook contributor Erin Zammett Ruddy has friends over for dinner, she invariably gets calls the next day asking for her recipes. But it's never for the pasta she slaved over or the expensive-ingredient desserts. It's always, always the salad dressing, the thing that took five minutes and a few shakes to throw together. This one calls for a whole chopped shallot, which gives the vinaigrette an oniony sweetness—the perfect complement to peppery arugula and bitter, tangy grapefruit.

Serves 2

1 bunch or bag (around 7 ounces) arugula
¼ cup red wine vinegar
½ teaspoon Dijon mustard
½ teaspoon sugar
1 shallot, minced
1 teaspoon coarse salt
½ teaspoon freshly ground black pepper
¾ cup extra-virgin olive oil
1 medium grapefruit, segmented (you can also buy segmented grapefruit in jars; if desired, substitute grapefruit with 2 tangerines or a blood orange)

1. Place the washed and dried arugula in a salad bowl; set aside.

2. In a small mixing bowl, whisk together the vinegar, mustard, sugar, shallot, salt, and pepper, then whisk in the olive oil.

3. Drizzle some of the dressing over the arugula and toss to coat. Top with the citrus segments and serve.

glamour girl tip

Every time Erin makes dressing, she doubles the recipe and keeps the extras in a Mason jar in the fridge for quick and easy salad assembly the rest of the week.

I Hang Out with Chefs Watermelon and Tomato Salad

Summery Salad of Watermelon, Tomatoes, Mint, and Almonds with Sherry Vinaigrette

Serves 4

DRESSING

2 tablespoons sliced almonds

3 garlic cloves, thinly sliced

Small squirt of Sriracha or other
   hot sauce

4 tablespoons extra-virgin olive oil

1 tablespoon sherry vinegar
   (or ½ tablespoon red wine/
   ½ tablespoon balsamic)

Juice of 1 lime

2 shallots, thinly sliced

Cookbook editor Veronica Chambers is pals with celebrity chef Marcus Samuelsson of New York's Red Rooster. Marcus has cooked for Veronica many times, but she's never cooked for *him* because, well, why would she? When your friend is the youngest chef to get three stars from the *New York Times*, it's a little intimidating! But when she's alone, Veronica does make Marcus's recipes—a lot. This one originally came from his book *New American Table*, but she's simplified it. The sweet chunks of watermelon are the perfect complement to the tangy tomatoes. When you toss in the almonds and capers, you've got what chefs call layers of flavor. We call it fabulous. Thanks, Marcus.

1. Make the vinaigrette: In a small skillet, combine the almonds, garlic, Sriracha, and 1 tablespoon olive oil and cook over moderate heat until toasted and fragrant, about 3 minutes. Remove from heat, and let cool.

2. In a small bowl, combine the remaining 3 tablespoons olive oil with the vinegar, lime juice, and shallots. Whisk in the cooled almond mixture.

3. Make the salad: In a large bowl, toss the watermelon, parsley, mint, capers, tomatoes, and vinaigrette to combine. Add salt and pepper to taste.

1 cup cubed watermelon
  (1-inch cubes)
2 tablespoons torn fresh flat-leaf
  parsley leaves
2 tablespoons torn fresh mint leaves
1 tablespoon capers, rinsed
3 red tomatoes, chopped into bite-size
  chunks
3 yellow tomatoes, chopped into
  bite-size chunks
Salt and freshly ground pepper

Serve This on a Big Plate Niçoise Salad

Mediterranean Salad with Eggs, Tuna, and Lemony Vinaigrette

Serves 3 to 4 as a lunchtime main course

SALAD

3 to 4 large eggs

1 pound green beans, ends trimmed

Salt

1 head lettuce (ideally romaine or
    red-leaf), coarsely chopped

Two 5-ounce cans tuna (olive
    oil–packed solid white tuna is best)

3 medium red potatoes, boiled and
    chopped (optional)

3 scallions, chopped

½ pint cherry tomatoes, halved

10 large fresh basil leaves, chopped,
    plus additional for garnish

4 anchovy fillets, quartered (optional)

½ cup olives, preferably kalamata,
    niçoise, or black olives, halved
    (optional)

Serving salad as a main course can be tricky; even the most health-conscious diner tends to see a plate of green and feel deprived. The secret to whipping up a hearty salad is adding protein (in this case, tuna) and letting good-for-you veggies like cherry tomatoes and green beans take the lead. "This salad behaves like a meal," says Anne Sachs, glamour.com's editorial director. She's right: The olives, scallions, and Dijon deliver salad-y flavor, but the tuna, potatoes, and eggs give it main-dish heft.

1. In a large saucepan, combine the eggs with enough cold water to cover by 2 inches. Bring to a boil, then turn the heat down to low and cook the eggs exactly 10 minutes. Carefully pour off the hot water, then shake the saucepan so the eggs bump onto each other to crack the shells. Run cold water over the eggs until they are cool enough to handle. Peel and quarter lengthwise.

2. Meanwhile, cook the green beans: Fill a skillet with 1 inch of water. Add ½ teaspoon salt, and simmer the beans over moderate heat for 7 to 8 minutes. Remove from the heat, drain, and let sit in a bowl of ice water for 5 minutes. Drain, then chop the beans in half and set aside.

3. Layer a medium or large salad platter with chopped lettuce, green beans, tuna, potatoes (if using), scallions, tomatoes, and basil. Layer the anchovy and/or olive pieces (if using) on top.

4. Prepare the dressing: Pour the olive oil into a small bowl and slowly whisk in the vinegar. Then whisk in the mustard, lemon juice, 1 teaspoon salt, and $\frac{1}{2}$ teaspoon pepper.

5. Just before serving, whisk the dressing again until well blended. Add the dressing to the bowl and toss well to coat, reserving extra dressing to store in the refrigerator (it will keep for a few days). Adjust the seasoning if necessary. Place the egg quarters decoratively across the top of the salad.

DRESSING

$\frac{3}{4}$ cup olive oil

$\frac{1}{4}$ cup red wine vinegar

$\frac{1}{4}$ teaspoon Dijon mustard

Juice of $\frac{1}{2}$ lemon

Freshly ground pepper

Please-a-Crowd Salad

Roasted Cherry Tomatoes, Spinach, and Gorgonzola Cheese Salad

Serves 6

SALAD

2 pints red or yellow cherry tomatoes

Olive oil for drizzling

Salt and freshly ground pepper

Leaves from 6 thyme sprigs

1 bag (around 10 ounces) washed baby
   spinach or arugula, torn into bite-size
   pieces

3 Belgian endives, thickly sliced

6 ounces Gorgonzola or other blue
   cheese

DRESSING

½ shallot, finely chopped

1 tablespoon Dijon mustard

Juice of 1 lemon

⅓ cup olive oil

Some days you're content just to bring a store-bought hummus platter to the potluck—but then there are those moments when your competitive spirit emerges and you want to bring Something Spectacular. This salad will do you proud: bright green spinach, red and yellow roasted cherry tomatoes, topped with restaurant-style shallot and mustard dressing. It's colorful and rich (and healthy, not that that's the point). You'll always go home with an empty bowl.

1. Preheat the oven to 450°F. Spread the tomatoes on a rimmed baking sheet lined with foil, and drizzle with olive oil. Season with salt, pepper, and thyme; toss the tomatoes gently to coat.

2. Roast the tomatoes for 15 minutes, or until almost bursting. (Check carefully during the last 5 minutes to avoid bursting; if any do burst, remove them from the pan with a slotted spoon.) Remove from the oven and let cool.

3. While the tomatoes are roasting, prepare the dressing: In a small bowl, combine the shallot, mustard, and lemon juice, and add a little salt and pepper. Whisk in ⅓ cup olive oil in a slow, steady stream.

4. In a salad bowl, combine the spinach, endives, and roasted tomatoes. Crumble the cheese over the salad and add the mustard-lemon dressing. Toss gently.

Workaholic's Salad

Stacked Tomato Salad with Polenta and Basil Vinaigrette

Serves 4 as a first course or
2 as a main

¼ cup fresh basil leaves

3 tablespoons olive oil, plus more for
brushing

Salt

2 large tomatoes, preferably heirloom
or vine ripened

Half a 16- to 18-ounce log ready-made
plain polenta, cut into four
½-inch-thick rounds

Freshly ground pepper

½ pound fresh mozzarella cheese,
cut into ¼-inch-thick slices

This vertical salad is beautiful enough to make anyone in your life who's had a long day at the office feel scrumptiously spoiled—hence its name. It's a twist on Caprese salad (tomato, mozzarella, basil) that gets stacked on top of a crisped polenta cake and drizzled with basil-specked oil for a surprisingly easy but truly impressive presentation. Using paper towels to absorb some of the liquid from the watery tomatoes is a genius step that ensures your stack won't be swimming in tomato juice. Polenta—an Italian ground cornmeal dish similar to grits—gives the salad enough substance to be dinner. Sit down, pour a glass of wine, and toast your favorite workaholic for a job well done.

1. In a blender, puree the basil with 3 tablespoons olive oil. Strain the puree through a very fine sieve into a bowl, pressing hard on the solids, then discard the solids. (Alternatively, skip the straining step and leave the minced basil in the oil.) Add ⅛ teaspoon salt to basil oil.

2. Cut the tomatoes crosswise into eight ½-inch-thick slices (slices cut from around the middle are best). Sandwich the slices between a triple layer of paper towels and press gently to remove any excess moisture.

3. Heat the grill, a grill pan, or medium skillet over moderately high heat. Generously brush both sides of the polenta rounds with olive oil, then add them to the grill. Cook, turning once, until lightly browned, about 5 minutes. Transfer one round to each plate.

4. Season the tomato slices with salt and pepper. Using a spatula, assemble 4 stacks by placing a tomato slice on top of each of the 4 polenta rounds. Top each with a mozzarella slice and another tomato slice. Drizzle basil oil over each stack before serving.

glamour girl tip

You can omit the polenta and end up with an elegant version of an Italian Caprese salad.

kitchen basics:
Six Ways to Make a Good Salad Better

1. Dry everything thoroughly. That's *especially* true for lettuce and herbs. Resist the impulse to cut corners—moisture on the leaves will cause wilting and keep the dressing from fully coating the greens. A salad spinner is worth the (not-so-high) price.

2. Use your hands. For most salads, there's no need to chop the lettuce with a knife. Tear it with your hands instead as you assemble; it will look more natural and have more compelling texture.

3. Chill it. To make your salad super-crispy, toss it with the dressing and put it in the freezer for 3 minutes before serving.

4. Add your fixings. Extras like golden raisins, sunflower seeds, avocado, or crumbled blue cheese make a salad more filling and delicious, and provide bonus nutrients.

5. Go nuts. For even more protein, flavor, and crunch, add crushed nuts like walnuts, almonds, or pecans. Or make Homemade Candied Nuts:

HOMEMADE CANDIED NUTS

1 tablespoon sugar
½ cup nuts (slivered almonds, sliced walnuts, or pecans work well)

1. Heat a small nonstick skillet over moderately high heat and add sugar. Watch the sugar closely so it doesn't burn, and stir it constantly with a wooden spoon once it starts to liquefy. When it's completely liquid, stir in nuts.

$2.$ Once the nuts start to turn brown but before they burn, scrape them onto wax paper or foil and let them cool completely.

$3.$ Break them up into little pieces and toss in with the salad.

$6.$ Dress it up. A good rule for vinaigrette is to use three parts oil to one part vinegar (although that balance can vary a bit, depending on the flavor of the olive oil and the kind of vinegar you use, not to mention the addition of other ingredients like mustard or herbs). Here are two of our favorite staples (these recipes make enough for several days' worth of salads; the dressings keep nicely in the fridge):

BASIC, JUST-RIGHT VINAIGRETTE

Whisk olive oil with vinegar in a glass or stainless steel bowl (an aluminum bowl will react with the acids in the vinegar). Add a dash of salt and pepper.

¾ cup olive oil (ideally extra-virgin)
¼ cup balsamic or red wine vinegar
Sea salt
Freshly ground black pepper

BASIC LEMON DRESSING

Whisk olive oil with lemon juice. Add a dash of salt and pepper, and blend in garlic.

½ cup olive oil (ideally extra-virgin)
½ cup freshly squeezed lemon juice
Sea salt
Freshly ground black pepper
1 garlic clove, minced (optional)

meat & poultry

Promotion Rib Eye

Seared Steaks Drizzled with Warm Butter

You know when you order steak in a restaurant and it's got that crusty sear on the outside and the inside is tender and buttery and you think, How come it doesn't turn out like this when *I* make it? Well, it's probably because you've never used this technique. Start by choosing the right cut of meat: a porterhouse, a strip steak, or— one of the best choices when you're in the mood to indulge—a rib eye. It's pricier, but packed with flavor, thanks to the marbling that runs throughout. A few cranks of salt and pepper is all the seasoning it needs. Then the trick is getting the pan super hot. *Hotter.* And finishing it in the oven, just like they do at restaurants. Consider it the perfect treat when you, or someone you love, done good.

Serves 2

Two 12- to 14-ounce boneless rib eye
   steaks, 1 to 1½ inches thick,
   at room temperature
Vegetable oil
Kosher salt and freshly ground black
   pepper
2 tablespoons butter (optional)

1. Preheat the oven to 500°F. Place a cast-iron skillet in the oven and preheat for 5 minutes. Using oven mitts, transfer the skillet to the stovetop and heat over moderately high heat. Turn the oven down to 450°F. (Remember that the handle of the skillet will be extremely hot when you take it out of the oven and will probably stay that way for a while.)

2. Coat the steaks liberally with oil and season well with salt and pepper. Place the steaks in the skillet (no additional oil is needed). Cook, turning once, until well charred, about 5 minutes.

[CONTINUED]

$3.$ Transfer the skillet to the 450°F oven and cook for about 4 minutes, turning once, until the meat is medium-rare and a meat thermometer inserted into the thickest part of the steak reads 125°F. Transfer the steaks to a plate and let rest for 5 to 7 minutes before serving. Optional: While you let the steaks rest, melt 2 tablespoons butter; drizzle the hot butter over the steak when it's ready to serve.

glamour girl tip

When cooking any kind of steak or burger, never push down on the meat—it forces the juices (and flavor) out. And always let meat rest for 5 to 7 minutes before cutting; that boosts the flavor too.

Prove to Mom You're Not Going to Starve Meat Loaf

Meat Loaf with Tomato Glaze

This is the perfect recipe to prep right before you call your parents on the phone. When they ask exactly what you're doing right this very second (because they love specifics, don't they?), casually offer, "Oh, just making a meat loaf." It will reassure them that you're a capital-G grown-up, and that maybe, just maybe, they can quit their worrying.

1. Preheat the oven to 375°F. Line a large rimmed baking sheet with parchment paper, and coat the paper with cooking spray. In a large skillet, heat 1 tablespoon olive oil. Add the onion, garlic, and bay leaf and cook over moderate heat, stirring a few times, until the onion is tender, about 6 minutes.

2. Add the bell pepper and cook, stirring occasionally, until tender, about 5 minutes. Stir in the parsley and thyme and cook for 2 minutes. Scrape the onion mixture into a bowl and let cool. Discard the bay leaf.

3. In a large bowl, combine the meat, egg, bread crumbs, 4 tablespoons ketchup, Worcestershire sauce, cayenne (if using), salt, pepper, and cooled onion-and-garlic mixture. Blend the ingredients with your hands. As soon as the ingredients are well combined, stop blending even if the mix isn't completely

Serves 3 to 4

Cooking spray
1 tablespoon olive oil
1 small yellow onion, diced
1 garlic clove, minced
1 bay leaf
½ medium red bell pepper, finely diced (about 1 cup)
1 tablespoon chopped fresh flat-leaf parsley
1 teaspoon chopped fresh thyme
1 pound lean ground beef or ground turkey (preferably dark meat)
1 large egg, lightly beaten
5 tablespoons dry bread crumbs
6 tablespoons ketchup
1½ teaspoons Worcestershire sauce
¼ teaspoon cayenne (optional)
1 teaspoon salt
½ teaspoon freshly ground black pepper

uniform. (Don't overwork the mixture or you'll risk ending up with a dry meat loaf.)

4. Transfer the meat mixture to the parchment-lined baking sheet and form it into a loaf. Alternatively, place the mixture in an 8- by 4-inch loaf pan to mold it, then turn it out onto the baking sheet. Coat the meat loaf with the remaining 2 tablespoons ketchup; if excess ketchup drips onto the parchment, wipe it off with a paper towel so it doesn't burn while the meat loaf is baking. Bake the meat loaf for about 1 hour, until the crust is richly browned and a meat thermometer inserted in the thickest part reads 165°F. Let it rest for 10 minutes before slicing. Serve.

glamour girl tip

Use any leftovers to make a terrific meat loaf sandwich: In a toaster oven or broiler, toast 2 slices of your favorite bread, arranging a few thin slices of Cheddar or mozzarella cheese on one side so they melt onto the bread. Then remove the bread from the toaster, spread the plain slice with mustard and a little ketchup, and top with a slice of meat loaf, a drizzle of olive oil, a few shreds of fresh basil leaves, and the second slice of bread.

Get Him to Clean the Apartment Burgers

Juicy Burgers on Toasted Buns

Nothing pleases after serious exertion like a burger. And if you don't have a grill, don't worry. You can get a similar "cooked on an open flame" effect by broiling these in the oven.

1. In a large bowl, using your hands, gently mix the meat with a generous pinch of salt, a few grinds of pepper, the cumin, shallot, and Worcestershire sauce, making sure not to take so long that you begin to warm the meat.

2. Divide into 2 balls (or 4 smaller balls) and flatten into patties.

3. With your thumbs, create a depression in the top and add a pat of butter to each patty. Refrigerate for 15 minutes.

4. Preheat the broiler or grill. If using the broiler, put the patties on a foil-lined rimmed baking sheet and broil for about 7 minutes, until they are browned on one side. Flip and cook for about 4 minutes longer, depending on how well done you like them. If using the grill, add the patties to the grill rack and cook over moderately high heat, turning once, until charred, about 7 minutes. If making cheeseburgers, add the cheese during the last few minutes of cooking.

Makes 2 large burgers or 4 smaller burgers

1 pound ground beef (80-to-20 meat-to-fat ratio—sorry, but leaner just won't do!)
Salt and freshly ground pepper
1 teaspoon ground cumin
1 shallot, finely chopped
2 dashes of Worcestershire sauce
2 to 4 pats (½ tablespoon each) butter
2 to 4 thin square slices Cheddar or Swiss cheese (optional)
2 to 4 hamburger buns, lightly toasted

[CONTINUED]

5. Place the burgers on the buns and add your favorite toppings. Close the burgers and serve.

VARIATION: TURKEY BURGERS

1 pound ground turkey

Generous pinch of salt

Multiple grinds of pepper

½ teaspoon ground cumin

1 shallot, finely chopped

1 tablespoon minced fresh oregano

1 tablespoon minced fresh cilantro

To make turkey burgers, substitute ground turkey (the fattiest available) for the ground beef. Reduce the cumin to ½ teaspoon, and replace the Worcestershire sauce with 1 tablespoon each minced fresh oregano and cilantro. If broiling, start watching the burgers after 5 minutes, turning them as soon as they are well browned. Before serving, cut into each burger to ensure that it is properly cooked through.

glamour girl tip

Whether turkey or beef, don't overhandle the meat—you want to leave pockets of air in the patties for the flavorful juices to collect.

No Guy Required Grilled Steak

Grilled Flank Steak Marinated in Ginger, Sesame, and Soy

You're a capable woman. You've negotiated raises, stared down your landlord, and endured the pain of brow tweezing and bikini waxing. The grill is *nothin'*, honey. This marinade, packed with flavor, is the perfect starter recipe. Just toss the dish together in the morning and pop it in the fridge. When you're ready to eat, fire up the grill (a grill pan works too) and in ten minutes you'll be in carnivore heaven.

Serves 2 to 3

One 1-pound flank steak
4 garlic cloves, minced
1 tablespoon minced fresh ginger or
⅛ tablespoon ground ginger
¼ cup soy sauce (reduced-sodium soy
sauce is fine)
¼ cup sugar
2 tablespoons fresh lime juice
Freshly ground pepper
1 tablespoon toasted sesame oil

1. Pat the steak dry with paper towels and make very light horizontal slits against the grain across both sides of the meat.

2. Transfer the steak to a large resealable plastic bag. Combine the garlic, ginger, soy sauce, sugar, lime juice, and pepper in a small bowl, then slowly whisk in the sesame oil until well blended. Pour the marinade over the steak and seal the bag, pushing out any excess air so the marinade surrounds the meat.

3. Refrigerate the meat for a minimum of 4 hours or up to 1 day, turning the bag 2 or 3 times.

[CONTINUED]

4. Light your grill (charcoal or gas), or if you're using a grill pan, preheat the broiler.

5. While grill is heating, remove steak from bag and pat dry. Transfer marinade to a small saucepan. Boil until thickened, about 3 minutes. Keep warm.

6. Once your grill is medium hot, place the steak on rack and grill for 6 to 8 minutes, turning once, until crisply browned and slightly charred on outside and medium-rare within. If steak is charring too quickly, move it to a cooler part of the grill. If you're using a grill pan, set the steak on it and broil for about 8 minutes, turning once, until charred and medium rare.

7. Allow the steak to rest for 10 minutes, then cut thin slices along the slits you made in step 1. (You should be cutting against the grain, at a 45-degree angle to the edge of the steak.) Serve with the cooked marinade.

a girl's guide to grilling

Step aside, boys! Your services are no longer needed. A basic guide for newbies from Diane Morgan, co-author of *Dressed to Grill* and author of *Grill Every Day*:

Preheat the grill. You should allow about 20 minutes for your grill to heat up, though charcoal grills take slightly longer. Try counting as you hold your hand over the grill until you can't stand it anymore. If you can only wait 2 seconds, the grill is very hot; if you can hold it for 5 seconds, the grill is around medium heat. The heat needed depends on what you're cooking, so check each recipe carefully. Don't make the mistake of grilling everything on high.

Arrange your food on the grill. If you're grilling a lot of food, start loading the grill from the back and move forward for easier manipulation. If you don't have a ton of food, keep the food toward the middle of the grill. Leave a cool spot on the grill so that you can move food around if you notice something is cooking too quickly.

WHEN YOU'RE GRILLING MEAT:

- Bring it to room temp. Grilling cold meat takes longer, so take the meat out of the fridge at least 20 (but no more than 60) minutes before grilling.

- Prep the meat. Pat it dry with paper towels. If meat has excess fat, trim it to about a quarter of an inch.

- Cook strategically. If you're grilling meat that needs to be cooked thoroughly on the inside (like chicken or pork), start by searing on high with the lid open. After the meat has nice grill marks, move it to the cooler part of the grill and shut the lid to capture the heat and finish cooking the meat. This ensures that your meat is cooked but the outside isn't torched.

WHEN YOU'RE GRILLING VEGGIES:

- Remember, size matters. Cut them about a half-inch thick, so they'll retain moisture and get nice grill marks, but won't fall through the grates.

- Keep an eye on them. Cooking times vary—vegetables can cook very quickly. Easiest to grill: peppers, asparagus, zucchini, and eggplant.

113

We're with the Band Moroccan Couscous

Moroccan Couscous with Lamb and Hot Pepper Sauce

Serves 4

2 tablespoons butter

1 pound boneless lamb shoulder or
   leg of lamb, cut into 1-inch cubes
   (ask your butcher to cube the lamb)

½ teaspoon salt

One ½-inch piece fresh ginger, peeled
   and minced

¼ teaspoon freshly ground black
   pepper

¼ teaspoon ground nutmeg

⅛ teaspoon turmeric

⅛ teaspoon ground cinnamon

1 whole clove

1½ cups chicken stock or water

1 large onion, chopped

2 carrots, cut into 1-inch pieces

2 medium zucchini, halved and cut
   into 1-inch pieces

⅓ cup raisins

½ cup canned chickpeas, drained

1 cup (8 ounces) cooked couscous

Tabasco, or your favorite hot pepper
   sauce

Morocco comes by its rock-and-roll legacy honestly. The Rolling Stones loved it, as did Jimi Hendrix and the Beatles. This Moroccan lamb couscous captures the vibe: It's exotic, but still jeans-and-black-leather-boots cool. Let your guests plop down on the floor on pillows to enjoy.

1. In a large stockpot, melt the butter over moderately high heat. Add the lamb and cook, turning occasionally, until browned, about 5 minutes. Stir in the salt, ginger, pepper, nutmeg, turmeric, cinnamon, and clove, stirring to coat the meat, and cook for 2 minutes, until fragrant.

2. Add the stock or water to the stockpot and bring to a boil. Turn the heat down to low, cover, and simmer for about 45 minutes, until the meat is just tender.

3. Add all the remaining ingredients except the couscous and hot pepper sauce; cover and cook 45 minutes longer, until the vegetables are tender.

4. Make the couscous according to the package directions. To serve, spoon the couscous and lamb into a warm serving dish. Serve with hot pepper sauce on the side.

Good Mood Tostadas

Crunchy Homemade Tostadas with Spicy Beef,
Cheddar Cheese, and Fresh Salsa

Traffic was crazy. Your hair had a mind of its own. The colleagues from hell were particularly hellish. Today just wasn't your day—but resist the urge to sit back with your good friends Ben & Jerry, and give these Good Mood Tostadas a try instead. Make sure the oil is super hot; that way, the tortillas will be in and out fast—the idea is to get them crisp and golden but not greasy. Then start layering and sprinkling the components on top like a Mexican pizza, and invite pals to share. Maybe it wasn't your day . . . but now it's your night.

1. Preheat the oven to 200°F. In a medium cast-iron skillet, heat 1 tablespoon oil over moderately high heat. Add the beef and cook, stirring to break up any lumps, until browned, about 6 minutes.

2. Spoon off any excess oil from the skillet. Stir in the taco seasoning and water and cook for 1 minute. Add salt to taste. Scrape the meat into a heatproof bowl, cover with foil, and keep warm in the oven. Wipe out the skillet.

3. Assemble the condiments in little bowls: diced onion, cilantro, lettuce, cheese, salsa, guacamole, and sour cream (if using).

[CONTINUED]

Serves 4 to 6

1 tablespoon vegetable oil, plus more
    for frying
1 pound ground beef
One 1¼-ounce package taco
    seasoning, or 1 teaspoon each
    ground cumin and chili powder
⅓ cup water
Salt
1 small red onion, diced
½ cup minced fresh cilantro
1½ cups shredded iceberg lettuce
1 cup grated Cheddar cheese
2 cups fresh salsa (page 53), or one
    16-ounce jar store-bought salsa
1 cup guacamole (optional; page 51)
1 cup sour cream (optional)
6 small corn tortillas (use flour tortillas
    if corn is not available)
One 16-ounce can refried beans,
    warmed in the microwave

4. Heat ½ inch of vegetable oil in the skillet over moderately high heat. Test the temperature of the oil: When a drop of water sizzles on the surface, using tongs, place 1 tortilla in the oil. Fry, turning once, until golden brown, about 1 minute. (A flour tortilla may bubble a bit, but it will flatten out after frying.) Transfer to a paper towel–lined plate. Repeat with the remaining tortillas.

5. To serve, spread each tostada with warm refried beans, then top with a few tablespoons of ground beef and the desired condiments.

glamour girl tip

It's always a good idea to buy extra ingredients when trying a new cooking technique, like frying tortillas. Tortillas usually come in packages of ten, so if you over- or undercook a few, you're still okay.

Instant Seduction Pork Chops

Juicy Ten-Minute Pork Chops with Rosemary and Thyme

This recipe comes from Jeff Mikkelson, a sexy photographer friend of ours (think Midwest farm boy meets downtown hipster) who loves to cook for the ladies in his life. "They say that the way to a man's heart is through his stomach, but I think that's the way to a *woman's* heart," he says. Jeff doesn't share the recipe with other men—"every guy has to work out his own game," he says—but we got him to spill the details for us. What makes this the perfect dinner à *deux* is the simple prep—you don't have to chop, sauté, or brown anything—and the easy cleanup. The makeshift tinfoil "dish" just gets tossed and you're done. Think your beloved could handle that? Flag this page, leave the cookbook lying around, and see.

Serves 2

1 tablespoon butter, plus more for
   greasing foil
Two ¾-inch-thick bone-in pork loin
   chops
2 garlic cloves, halved
Salt and freshly ground pepper
1 teaspoon dried oregano
1 teaspoon dried thyme
A few rosemary sprigs

1. Preheat the broiler. Roll out a double-layer piece of aluminum foil large enough to hold both chops (roughly 12 inches square) and turn up the edges to create a "pan." Coat the surface of the foil with butter. (The easiest way to do this is to smear the exposed edge of a stick of butter all over the foil.)

2. Place the pork chops on the foil, and rub them all over with the cut sides of the garlic cloves, 1 garlic clove half per side of the chops. Using a sharp paring knife, make 2 slits in each chop, and slide half a garlic clove into each slit.

[CONTINUED]

3. Sprinkle each chop generously on both sides with salt, pepper, oregano, thyme, and rosemary. Place a thin pat of butter (about ½ tablespoon) on each chop, and place the chops on the foil pan under the broiler, about 4 inches from the heat.

4. Broil the chops for 5 minutes on one side, then turn over and broil for 3 to 5 minutes, until they reach the desired doneness. Transfer the pork chops to a plate, pour the juices from the foil pan on top, and let rest for a few minutes before serving. (You can either leave the cloves in or, if you're not a garlic fan, remove them.)

glamour girl tip

Depending on the thickness of your chop, you may want to stick to the low end of the suggested cooking times. Most people are afraid to eat their pork a little pink, but it's actually okay to cook it to just 160°F—and it's much more tender and flavorful that way.

Man Salad

Marinated Skirt Steak Salad with Arugula

Forget the whole only-women-love-salad cliché. Skirt steak with a salty-sweet glaze sliced on top of peppery arugula with earthy mushrooms: How could anyone—even the most guy-ish of guys—not want *that*?

Serves 2

1 garlic clove
½ teaspoon kosher or sea salt
1½ tablespoons fresh lemon juice
1 tablespoon soy sauce
2 teaspoons sugar
1 pound skirt steak, cut in 2 pieces
1 teaspoon olive oil
5 large mushrooms, cut into wedges
½ red bell pepper, cut into strips
½ small red onion, thinly sliced
5 ounces arugula (or 1 small head
   green leaf lettuce)

1. Mince the garlic and mash with the salt to make a paste. Put in a small bowl and stir in the lemon juice, soy sauce, and sugar.

2. Put the steak in a large resealable plastic bag and add about two-thirds of the garlic-soy mixture. Remove the air from the bag and seal, then massage the meat to coat with the marinade. Let stand at room temperature for 10 minutes, or refrigerate for up to 2 hours.

3. Heat a 10-inch cast-iron skillet over moderately high heat until hot, at least 2 minutes. Add the oil, swirling to coat the pan, and add the steak. Cook on each side, without moving, until browned, about 3 minutes per side for medium-rare. Transfer the steaks to a plate to rest, then add the mushrooms and red pepper to the skillet and cook over moderate heat until softened slightly, about 3 minutes.

[CONTINUED]

4. Toss the onion and lettuce in a bowl with enough of the remaining garlic-soy mixture to coat, then arrange the salad on two plates. Slice the steak crosswise on an angle and arrange on top of the salad. Top with the mushrooms and red pepper.

VARIATION: STEAK SANDWICH

Turn the salad into steak sandwiches: Halve a French baguette crosswise, then lengthwise for 2 sandwiches. Fill with the salad, steak, and cooked vegetables.

Too Hot to Cook Turkey Tonnato

Turkey Breast with Italian-Style Tuna and Caper Sauce

Need an easy dish for a seriously steamy summer day? *Glamour* editor-in-chief Cindi Leive recommends this clever, no-cook turkey dish, one of her favorite recipes from her dog-eared copy of *Glamour's Gourmet on the Run*. It's a riff on the Italian classic vitello tonnato, but it calls for deli-counter turkey instead of veal, so it's inexpensive and easy to pull off. The creamy, rich tuna-anchovy sauce gets whirred together in a food processor and spooned on top. Cindi first made it for a friend's bridal shower and it got rave reviews; it's still in her repertoire. Serve it alongside greens topped with ricotta salata or feta cheese.

Serves 4

1 pound sliced roasted turkey breast

1 cup mayonnaise

One 5-ounce can tuna, drained

One third 2-ounce can flat anchovies, drained (2 anchovies)

1½ tablespoons fresh lemon juice, plus 1 lemon, sliced, for garnish

¼ teaspoon paprika

1½ tablespoons capers, rinsed

1. Arrange the turkey slices on a platter.

2. In a blender or food processor, mix the mayonnaise, tuna, anchovies, lemon juice, paprika, and 1 tablespoon capers. Add more lemon juice to taste, if necessary. Spoon the sauce over the turkey.

3. Garnish with the remaining ½ tablespoon capers and lemon slices and serve.

Fight Over It Fried Chicken

Fried Chicken with Paprika and Cayenne

Serves 2

Vegetable oil for frying (about 8 cups)

½ teaspoon freshly ground black
  pepper

½ teaspoon garlic powder

1 teaspoon salt

4 chicken pieces with skin, such as
  breast halves, thighs, or legs

1 cup all-purpose flour

1 teaspoon paprika, preferably hot
  smoked

1 teaspoon cayenne

Glamour senior editor Leslie Robarge is an expert cook—but even experts have mishaps. The first time she made fried chicken with her best friend for a dinner party, things didn't go as well as they had hoped. They'd planned on serving their ten guests at 8:00 P.M., but it took three more hours, ten bottles of wine, and a hearty helping of bourbon before they finally brought out the finished product. Everyone was so excited (and a little tipsy) that they clapped, Leslie laughed, and her platter went flying to the floor—at which point the guests dove for the chicken and gobbled it down anyway.

Glamour has altered the recipe to cut the time (if cooking for a group, use two pans), but did nothing to change the taste of a dish so good that guests are perfectly willing to eat it off the floor.

1. In a 4-inch-deep heavy pot or deep fryer fitted with a thermometer, heat 2 inches of oil to 350°F. (If you don't have a thermometer, drop a kernel of popcorn into the oil; the kernel will pop when the oil is hot enough—in the 350°F to 365°F range.)

2. Meanwhile, mix together the black pepper, garlic powder, and ½ teaspoon salt. Pat the chicken dry, then sprinkle all over with the pepper mixture.

3. Put the flour, paprika, cayenne, and remaining ½ teaspoon salt in a large plastic bag, then seal the bag and toss to mix the ingredients. Put the chicken pieces in the bag, then reseal. Toss to coat the chicken evenly.

4. Fry the breasts first in the oil, turning as necessary, until evenly browned and cooked through, 12 to 15 minutes. Drain the chicken on a plate lined with paper towels. Return the oil to 350°F and cook the legs, thighs, and/or drumsticks until evenly browned and cooked through, 15 to 18 minutes. Drain on a plate lined with paper towels and serve.

kitchen basics:

Five $5 Chicken Dinners

Boneless, skinless chicken breasts—so wonderfully affordable, yet so dull if they're not prepared the right way. Here are five fantastically tasty recipes for chicken breasts, and none of them will run you much more than $5 a serving. Each recipe serves 2.

2 chicken breasts
Salt and freshly ground
   pepper

To start: Keep a bag of individually wrapped boneless, skinless chicken breasts in your freezer, and thaw them in the fridge during the day or overnight, as microwave defrosting can turn edges tough. Before cooking, pound each between two sheets of plastic wrap or wax paper (using the flat side of a cleaver, rolling pin, or meat pounder if you have one) until they're ¼-inch thick. Sprinkle each pounded chicken breast with ½ teaspoon salt and ¼ teaspoon freshly ground pepper, making sure to season both sides. Each recipe below calls for 2 chicken breasts.

CHICKEN PROVENÇAL

1. Evenly coat each chicken breast with 1 tablespoon flour.

2. Heat olive oil and butter in a 12-inch skillet over moderate heat, then cook the chicken until lightly golden, 2 minutes per side. Transfer the chicken to a plate.

3. In the skillet, add fennel bulb, onion, garlic, and herbes de Provence or dried thyme. Cook over moderate heat, stirring occasionally, until the fennel and onion have softened, 2 to 3 minutes.

4. Add white wine and bring to a boil. Add tomatoes, olives, and the chicken, then cover and simmer until the chicken is cooked through, 10 minutes.

5. Stir in parsley and serve.

2 tablespoons flour
1 tablespoon olive oil
1 tablespoon unsalted butter
1 cup thinly sliced fennel bulb
½ cup sliced onion
1 large garlic clove, minced
1 teaspoon herbes de Provence or dried thyme
¾ cup dry white wine
½ cup canned diced tomatoes
¼ cup dry-cured black olives
2 tablespoons chopped fresh flat-leaf parsley

ITALIAN CHICKEN

1. Coarsely chop pancetta, then cook in a 12-inch skillet over moderate heat, stirring occasionally, until browned. Remove the pancetta from the pan with a slotted spoon and reserve. Leave the rendered fat in the skillet.

2. Evenly coat each breast with 2 tablespoons flour.

3. Add butter to the fat in the skillet, then cook the chicken over moderate heat until lightly golden, 2 minutes per side. Transfer the chicken to a plate.

2 ounces pancetta
4 tablespoons flour
1 tablespoon unsalted butter
½ cup sliced onion
6 ounces marinated artichokes (drained and cut in half lengthwise)
½ teaspoon finely chopped fresh rosemary
1 garlic clove, minced

1 cup dry white wine (such
　　as sauvignon blanc or
　　pinot grigio)
1 tablespoon chopped fresh
　　flat-leaf parsley
2 tablespoons freshly grated
　　Parmigiano-Reggiano
　　cheese

4. In the skillet, add onion, artichokes, and rosemary and cook, stirring occasionally, until the onion has softened, 2 to 3 minutes. Add garlic and cook 1 minute more. Add white wine and bring to a boil.

5. Add the chicken to the skillet, then cover and simmer until it is cooked through, 10 minutes. Stir in the pancetta and parsley.

6. To serve, spoon the artichoke mixture over the chicken breasts and sprinkle each with 1 tablespoon cheese.

ASIAN CHICKEN

2 tablespoons flour
3 tablespoons vegetable oil
4 ounces shiitake mush-
　　rooms, stemmed and
　　thinly sliced
2 scallions, chopped
1 teaspoon grated fresh
　　ginger
1 garlic clove, minced
Red pepper flakes
1 cup chicken stock
½ teaspoon soy sauce
¼ teaspoon sesame oil
¼ cup chopped fresh
　　cilantro
¼ cup chopped scallions

1. Evenly coat each piece of chicken with 1 tablespoon flour.

2. Heat 2 tablespoons vegetable oil in a 12-inch skillet over moderate heat, and cook the chicken until lightly golden, 2 minutes per side. Transfer the chicken to a plate.

3. Add 1 tablespoon oil to the pan. Cook mushrooms, scallions, ginger, garlic, and a pinch of red pepper flakes over moderate heat, stirring occasionally, until the scallions and mushrooms begin to soften, 2 to 3 minutes.

4. Add chicken stock, soy sauce, sesame oil, and the chicken, then cover and simmer until the chicken is cooked through, 10 minutes.

5. Serve the chicken with the sauce spooned over, and top with cilantro and scallions.

BISTRO-STYLE CHICKEN WITH RED WINE

1. Evenly coat each piece of chicken with 1 table-spoon flour.

2. Heat butter in a 12-inch skillet over moderate heat, then cook the chicken until lightly golden, 2 minutes per side. Transfer the chicken to a plate.

3. In the skillet, add onion, mushrooms, and thyme. Cook until the onion and mushrooms have softened, about 5 minutes. Add garlic and cook, stirring, 1 minute more.

4. Stir in red wine and tomato paste. Add bacon, then the chicken. Cover and simmer until just cooked through, 10 minutes.

5. Serve each piece sprinkled with parsley.

2 tablespoons flour
2 tablespoons unsalted
  butter
1 cup sliced onion
4 ounces sliced mushrooms
½ teaspoon dried thyme
1 garlic clove, minced
1 cup full-bodied red wine
  (such as cabernet
  sauvignon, zinfandel, or
  merlot)
1 tablespoon tomato paste
2 ounces diced bacon
1 tablespoon chopped fresh
  flat-leaf parsley

MEXICAN CHICKEN

1. Evenly coat each piece of chicken with 1 table-spoon flour.

2. Heat olive oil in a 12-inch skillet over moderate heat, and cook the chicken until lightly golden, 2 minutes per side. Transfer the chicken to a plate.

3. In the skillet, add onion, jalapeño, cumin, and oregano, and cook over moderate heat, stirring occasionally, until the onion has softened, 2 to 3 minutes. Add chicken stock and white wine and bring to a boil.

2 tablespoons flour
2 tablespoons olive oil
1 cup chopped onion
1 fresh jalapeño pepper,
  finely chopped
½ teaspoon ground cumin
½ teaspoon dried oregano
½ cup chicken stock
¼ cup dry white wine (such
  as sauvignon blanc or
  pinot grigio)

½ firm ripe avocado, sliced

2 tablespoons sour cream

4 tablespoons chopped
fresh cilantro

2 to 4 lime wedges, for
serving

4. Add the chicken, cover, and simmer until the chicken is cooked though, 10 minutes.

5. To serve, spoon the sauce over the chicken, then top each piece of chicken with avocado, sour cream, and cilantro. Serve with a wedge or two of lime on the side.

seafood

Simply Sophisticated Seared Tuna

Tuna Steaks Seared with Ginger, Soy, and Brown Sugar

Glamour.com assistant editor Meredith Turits calls this her go-to dish anytime she wants to make something easy and impressive. It gets her lots of looks that say: Who knew *you* went to culinary school? Serve with Beyond Basic Broccoli (page 192) and rice.

Serves 2

1 tablespoon peeled and minced fresh ginger

1 garlic clove, minced

2 tablespoons brown sugar

¼ cup soy sauce

2 tablespoons fresh lemon juice

Two 6-ounce tuna steaks, about ¾-inch thick

Salt and freshly ground pepper

1 tablespoon olive oil

2 scallions, thinly sliced

1. In a deep dish or pie plate, mix the ginger, garlic, brown sugar, soy sauce, and lemon juice. Stir until combined.

2. Season the tuna generously with salt and pepper on both sides. Place the tuna in the dish with the marinade and turn to coat. Cover and refrigerate for 1 hour, turning the fish at least once.

3. In a large cast-iron skillet, heat 1 tablespoon oil over moderate heat.

4. Remove the tuna from the marinade, pat dry, and add the steaks to the skillet. Cook, turning once, until browned and just cooked through, about 8 minutes total. Transfer to plates and sprinkle with scallions. Serve. (If desired, heat the remaining marinade in a small saucepan and boil for 2 minutes, then serve with the tuna.)

glamour girl tip

If you have a grill pan, this fish can be cooked for about 3 minutes on each side.

Bikini Season Baked Salmon

Salmon with Lemon, White Wine, and Capers

Serves 4

Four 8-ounce skin-on salmon fillets
Sea salt and freshly ground pepper
3 tablespoons olive oil
½ cup dry white wine
½ cup chopped fresh flat-leaf parsley
½ cup fresh lemon juice
2 tablespoons capers

Yes, salmon is good for you. It's jam-packed with heart-healthy omega-3s, which can actually help your body burn fat more efficiently. But the real reason this recipe is so figure-friendly is that it's so easy you'll happily make and eat it once a week. (Leftovers can get chopped over greens for a salad, or mixed with lemon juice and capers for a yummy sandwich filling.)

1. Preheat the oven to 400°F. Put the salmon skin-side down in a ceramic or glass baking pan. Rub the salmon fillets with 1 tablespoon olive oil and season generously with salt and pepper. Let the salmon sit in the pan for 10 minutes.

2. Drizzle the white wine over the salmon, then sprinkle ¼ cup parsley on top; save the remaining parsley to use later. Put the pan in the oven and cook for 15 to 20 minutes, or until the salmon fillets are opaque.

3. Meanwhile, in a small bowl, mix the lemon juice, capers, remaining parsley, and 2 tablespoons olive oil. Top each salmon fillet with the lemon juice mixture and serve immediately.

Can We Talk? Crab Cakes

Maryland-Style Crab Cakes with Basil Mayonnaise

When *Glamour* editorial assistant Jessica Duncan was growing up in Georgia, she practically lived in her mother's kitchen. Not just because her mom, Vickie Myers, is a great cook, but because she's a great listener. Vickie would whip up a batch of her famous crab cakes (using crabs caught by her husband in the river behind their house!) while Jessica talked. The prep takes a while—about 45 minutes—so there's ample time to catch up on everything. This is the perfect dinner for a leisurely evening with people you love—and enjoy listening to.

1. Fill a medium saucepan with water. Add a large pinch of salt and bring to a boil. Add the basil and cook over high heat for 30 seconds (this quick plunge in boiling water is called blanching). Drain. Immediately transfer the leaves to a large bowl of ice water. Drain, wiping out the bowl. Pat the basil dry with paper towels. Finely chop the basil.

2. In the bowl, mix the mayonnaise, mustard, lemon juice, and cayenne. Set aside ½ cup of the mayonnaise mixture to use when preparing the crab cakes. Stir the basil into the remaining mayonnaise, and refrigerate the basil mayonnaise to serve with the crab cakes when they're ready.

[CONTINUED]

Makes 6 to 8 crab cakes; serves 3 to 4

BASIL MAYONNAISE
Salt
40 fresh whole basil leaves
1½ cups mayonnaise
2 teaspoons Dijon mustard
2 teaspoons fresh lemon juice
¼ teaspoon cayenne

CRAB CAKES
1 pound fresh lump crabmeat, picked free of shells
½ cup reserved mayonnaise mixture
¼ cup chopped fresh chives
2 tablespoons fresh chopped flat-leaf parsley
2⅔ cups dry white bread crumbs
6 tablespoons olive or vegetable oil
2 celery stalks, finely chopped
⅔ cup finely chopped onion
Salt and freshly ground pepper
¼ cup plus 2 tablespoons all-purpose flour
3 large eggs

3. In a large bowl, carefully stir together the crabmeat, reserved mayonnaise mixture, chives, parsley, and $^2/_3$ cup of bread crumbs, making sure not to break the crab up too much.

4. In a large, heavy skillet, heat 2 tablespoons oil over moderate heat. Add the celery and onion and cook, stirring a few times, until tender, about 5 minutes. Transfer to a plate and let cool slightly, then add the celery-onion mixture to the crab mixture and gently combine. Season to taste with salt and pepper.

5. Form the crab mixture into 6 to 8 cakes. Refrigerate for at least 20 minutes, until the cakes are firm. (Don't skip this step; the chilling keeps them from falling apart as they cook.)

6. Place the flour in a small bowl. In another small bowl, whisk the eggs to blend them together. Place the remaining 2 cups bread crumbs in a medium bowl. Line the bowls up next to each other so you can easily dip the crab cakes into one after the other.

7. Heat 2 tablespoons oil in a large skillet over moderate heat. Working in two batches, remove half the crab cakes from the refrigerator. Working with one crab cake at a time, coat each one with flour, then dip into the beaten egg, then coat completely with bread crumbs. Add the crab cakes to the hot skillet and cook, turning once, until golden and crisp, about 5 minutes. Using a spatula, transfer the crab cakes to a plate. Add another 2 tablespoons oil to the skillet and repeat the process with the second batch. These can be made ahead and refrigerated until ready to serve. Reheat for 10 to 15 minutes in an oven preheated to 350°F. Serve with basil mayonnaise.

Season Finale Shrimp

Steamed Shrimp in Beer with Lemon, Garlic, and Butter

You've invited your friends over to watch an episode, maybe the last episode ever, of your favorite show. You want finger food, and—since you don't want to miss a second of screen time—you want a quick recipe. This dish only takes ten minutes to throw together—you literally toss all the ingredients into a pot. We like to serve our guests ice-cold bottles of the same kind of beer we used to steam the shrimp. When an ingredient makes two very different appearances in a meal, chefs call it bridging; we call it fun, and frugal!

Serves 4

1 pound large shrimp (fresh or frozen), cleaned, shelled, and deveined

1 bay leaf

6 dill sprigs or 1 teaspoon dill weed

1 garlic clove, minced

Juice of ½ lemon

½ teaspoon salt

¼ teaspoon whole peppercorns

⅛ teaspoon dried red pepper flakes

1 cup beer

¼ cup butter, melted (optional)

1. In a large saucepan, combine all the ingredients except the butter, and bring to a boil.

2. Immediately cover the saucepan, remove from heat, and let stand 4 to 6 minutes, or until the shrimp are pink and curl up. Drain and transfer the shrimp to a plate. Discard the bay leaf, dill, and garlic.

3. Serve the shrimp hot with melted butter for dipping, if you like.

Beach House Grilled Shrimp

Shrimp with Fresh Corn, Tomatoes, and Basil

Serves 4 as an appetizer or
2 as a main course

16 large tail-on shrimp, cleaned,
    shelled, and deveined
6 tablespoons olive oil
1 garlic clove, minced
3 ears corn, shucked
2 cups chopped tomatoes (or grape
    tomatoes, halved, if good tomatoes
    are not in season)
8 basil leaves, finely chopped
Salt and freshly ground pepper
Lime wedges, for serving (optional)

Woo-hoo! You're going to the shore! Or maybe you're not, but so what? This recipe—showcasing some of summer's greatest hits: corn, tomatoes, and basil—will bring the beach vibe to you. Buy the veggies fresh and you won't have to add more than a drizzle of olive oil and a sprinkle or two of salt and pepper; they're that tasty.

1. In a large bowl, toss the shrimp (tails on!) with 3 table-spoons olive oil and the minced garlic; marinate 30 minutes.

2. Meanwhile, bring a large pot of salted water to a boil. Add the corn and cook over high heat for about 4 minutes. Drain and let cool under running water. Using a large serrated knife and working over a large bowl with one ear at a time, cut the kernels from the cobs by standing each ear of corn upright in the bowl and carefully running the edge of the knife vertically down each side, cutting close to the cob; the kernels will fall off the cob and into the bowl.

3. Add the tomatoes, basil, and 2 tablespoons olive oil to the bowl with the corn and toss well. Add salt and pepper to taste.

4. Remove the shrimp from the marinade and season with salt and pepper. In a large skillet, heat the remaining 1 tablespoon of olive oil over moderately high heat. Add the shrimp and cook until just white throughout, about 4 minutes. Using tongs or a slotted spoon, transfer the shrimp to the bowl with the corn mixture and toss. Serve with lime wedges for squeezing on top, if desired.

Skinny Jeans Scallops

Mediterranean-Style Scallops with Olives and Oregano

Serves 4

SCALLOPS

2 tablespoons olive oil

1 tablespoon red wine vinegar

1 garlic clove, finely chopped

2 teaspoons finely chopped fresh
    oregano

1½ pounds large sea scallops (about
    20), cleaned

SAUCE

2 tablespoons extra-virgin olive oil

2 celery stalks, diced into ¼-inch
    cubes

1 garlic clove, minced

2 ripe tomatoes, cut into ¼-inch dice

¼ cup kalamata or other brine-cured
    black olives, pitted and coarsely
    chopped

2 tablespoons small capers, drained
    and chopped

3 tablespoons chopped fresh flat-leaf
    parsley

3 tablespoons finely chopped fresh
    basil

No need to count calories when you're making a dish as light and satisfying as this. It has Italian spirit—thanks to the olives, capers, and tomatoes—and marinating the scallops before searing lets those flavors soak through. There you go! A "diet" that doesn't taste it. So *that's* how those European ladies do it.

1. In a large resealable plastic bag, combine the oil, vinegar, garlic, oregano, and scallops. Close the bag and seal it tightly, pressing out the excess air. Refrigerate for 20 minutes, turning occasionally.

2. Make the sauce: In a large heavy skillet, heat the oil over medium heat until hot. Add the celery and cook, stirring, until tender, about 4 minutes. Increase the heat to moderately high and add the garlic, tomatoes, 2 tablespoons water, olives, and capers and cook until the sauce is slightly thickened, about 5 minutes.

3. Stir in the parsley, basil, vinegar, salt, and pepper. Cover and remove from the heat.

4. Remove the scallops from the bag and shake off any excess marinade. Lightly oil a grill pan or cast-iron skillet and

heat over moderately high heat until smoking. Grill the scallops, turning once, until just cooked through, about 5 minutes.

5. Spoon the sauce over the scallops. Serve over rice or orzo, if desired.

glamour girl tip

The sauce is also delicious spooned over a white fish like cod and halibut or shrimp.

1 tablespoon red wine vinegar

¼ teaspoon salt

¼ teaspoon freshly ground black pepper

Cooked rice or orzo, for serving (optional)

Perfect Host Lobster Pot Pie

Seriously Loaded Shellfish-Stuffed Pastry

Serves 4

8 tablespoons unsalted butter (1 stick)

1½ cups chopped yellow onion (about
   1 large onion)

1 cup chopped celery

½ cup all-purpose flour

2 tablespoons white wine

2½ cups fish stock or vegetable stock

Salt and freshly ground pepper

¼ cup heavy cream

1 pound cooked lobster meat, roughly
   chopped

1½ cups frozen corn, not thawed

1½ cups frozen pearl onions,
   not thawed

½ cup coarsely chopped fresh
   flat-leaf parsley

2 refrigerated premade pie crusts

1 large egg beaten with 2 tablespoons
   water

This decadent recipe—another Veronica Chambers invention—is shockingly easy. It calls for canned lobster, premade pie crust, and a filling that takes less than 30 minutes. Whenever Veronica makes this, she likes to make two: one for dinner and one for her guests to take home. In the summer, they are luxurious vacation-worthy fare, even when served in a small landlocked apartment. In the winter, these lobster pot pies are warm and comforting, and make you dream of summer. They also freeze beautifully. And in individual ramekins (see Variation), you—good host that you are—can send friends home with any that are left over.

1. Preheat the oven to 375°F. In a large skillet, heat the butter over moderate heat. Once melted, add the onion and celery and cook, stirring a few times, until the onion is translucent, about 10 minutes.

2. Turn the heat down to low, sprinkle the flour over the onion mixture, and stir to combine. Cook, stirring occasionally, for 3 minutes longer. Add white wine and cook for 1 minute.

3. Add the stock, 1 teaspoon salt, and ½ teaspoon pepper and simmer for 5 minutes. Pour in the heavy cream.

4. In a large bowl, combine lobster, frozen corn and onions, and parsley, and add salt and pepper to taste. Pour liquid mixture over lobster mixture. Stir and set aside. Unroll one premade pie crust in a dish and fill with the lobster mixture. Top with the second pie crust. Crimp the edges together and brush with the egg wash. Make 4 or 5 slashes on top of the crust and bake for 1 hour and 15 minutes, until the top is golden brown and the filling is bubbling.

VARIATION: PERSONAL POT PIES

To make individual lobster pot pies: Unroll the pie dough and, with a sharp knife, cut it into circles to fit four 5- to 6-ounce individual ramekins or other ovenproof bowls. Line each ramekin with the circle of dough, fill with the lobster mixture, and top with another cutout circle of pie dough. Crimp the edges together, brush each pie with egg wash, and follow the remaining instructions above. Cook for 50 minutes and then check. Pot pies are done when the tops are golden brown.

kitchen basics:
What You Need to Know About Seafood

It's delicious, nutritious…and, if you're new to cooking it, frankly intimidating. These tips should help you feel confident:

WHEN YOU SHOP:

- Smell the fish. All seafood should smell like an ocean breeze; it should not have an unpleasantly fishy smell.

- Look closely. Fin fish (which means every fish but shellfish) should be slightly translucent and have a moist, glossy look. The flesh should feel firm and spring back when you press it. If you're buying whole fish, any scales should be firmly attached and the eyes should be bright and bulging, not brown, milky, or sunken. If you're buying a cut of fish, like a steak or fillet, the flesh should never appear dry or brownish at the edges. Shellfish like shrimp or scallops should have a firm texture. Oysters, mussels, or clams should be tightly closed. Cooked lobster meat or crabmeat should be white with a reddish tinge.

WHEN YOU COOK:

- Sautéing works best for relatively small fish fillets like flounder, sole, or tilapia. In a large skillet, heat a small amount of butter or oil (about 1 tablespoon) over moderately high heat. Add the fish fillets and cook for about 3 to 4 minutes per side. Season with salt, pepper, and fresh lemon juice, then sprinkle with minced fresh herbs like basil or fresh flat-leaf parsley.

- Baking is a safe choice for thicker fish steaks like salmon or swordfish and thicker fillets like grouper and cod. Preheat the oven to 350°F. Grease a baking pan with butter or oil, then coat the fish with olive oil and sprinkle each piece with salt and pepper, 1 teaspoon lemon juice, and 1 teaspoon white wine. Bake for 8 to 10 minutes per inch of thickness. Serve with lemon wedges.

- Broiling is fantastic for virtually any kind of fish, especially fillets or steaks. Preheat the broiler. Coat the fish with olive oil or melted butter; drizzle each piece with 1 teaspoon lemon juice and, if desired, 1 teaspoon white wine, and sprinkle with salt and pepper. Broil in a broiling pan, without a rack, about 3 to 4 inches from the heat source, for 8 to 10 minutes per inch of thickness. Don't turn the fish as it broils. Sprinkle minced fresh flat-leaf parsley on top, or garnish with capers and serve with wedges of lemon.

- Grilling is good for thicker types of fish, like tuna or salmon; thinner cuts will fall apart. To grill more delicate fish, wrap it in foil. Preheat your grill as hot as it can go, then cook the fish for 5 to 7 minutes per inch of thickness, flipping once halfway through and watching it closely to be sure it doesn't scorch. Some fish, like tuna, can be served rare and just needs a nice sear on the grill before it's ready to go. All you need is a squirt of lemon juice and a dash of salt and pepper.

AND IF YOU'RE CONCERNED ABOUT SAFETY...

Headlines about toxins, mercury, and the environment have us all worried. Your best bets are salmon, shrimp, canned light tuna, and pollock; these fish have lower levels of mercury. Try to avoid swordfish, king mackerel, tilefish (also known as golden bass or golden snapper), and shark because they have higher mercury levels. Follow this rule of thumb: the smaller the fish, the better. And remember, fish is a great source of protein and omega-3 fatty acids, so you don't need to—and shouldn't—avoid it altogether. If you have safety questions, visit fda.gov and epa.gov for information.

pizza
&
pasta

Perfect Date Night Pizza

Basic Pizza Pie Dough, with Topping Variations

Our friend Klancy Miller trained as a pastry chef at Le Cordon Bleu in Paris, so when she told us that making our own pizza dough would be easy, we suspected that *her* easy might not be the same as *our* easy. But we've since come around. Klancy believes that making pizza is the perfect date night activity. You start the dough and then you've got an hour while it rises. Do what you like with that hour. (You two can fill the time, can't you?) Then return to the dough, finish up the pizza, and chow down.

Alternatively, you can make this pizza with premade dough, eliminating the hour wait. (Look for balls of dough in the dairy section or the frozen pizza aisle.) But don't be afraid to try the homemade version at least once: It surprised every one of our testers with its ease.

Makes 1 pizza; serves 4

DOUGH

One ¼-ounce package active dry yeast

½ cup warm water (105° to 115°F)

1⅔ cups all-purpose flour, plus more for sprinkling

1 teaspoon salt

1 tablespoon olive oil, plus more for oiling the dough

BASIC PIZZA PIE DOUGH

1. In a small bowl, cover the yeast with the warm water. Let stand 5 minutes to activate, then stir to dissolve. In a large bowl, combine the flour and salt and form a well in the center (as though the flour were mashed potatoes and you're making room for gravy).

2. Pour the yeast mixture and the tablespoon of oil into the well, then gradually work the liquids into the flour with a fork until a loose dough forms. If the dough seems too sticky, mix

in a sprinkling of additional flour; if it seems too stiff, add a sprinkling of water. The dough should be supple and smooth.

3. Transfer the dough to a lightly floured surface and knead for 10 minutes, sprinkling with flour as needed, until the dough is lump-free. Rub oil over the dough and return it to the bowl.

4. Cover with plastic wrap and let rise at room temperature for about 1 hour, until the dough has doubled in bulk. Transfer to a lightly floured surface and knead for 30 seconds longer. If not making pizza right away, keep the dough in a resealable plastic bag in the fridge for up to 24 hours, or freeze until ready to use.

5. When ready to make a pizza, using your fingers or a rolling pin, roll out or press the dough to the desired size. (For minimal fuss, instead of striving for a perfect circle, you can put the dough directly on a lightly oiled rimmed baking sheet and press to fit with your fingertips, making sure to push it all the way into the corners.)

6. Add any of the topping variations below, or your own favorite pizza toppings.

CLASSIC TOMATO SAUCE

Makes enough sauce for 1 pizza

3 tablespoons olive oil
3 garlic cloves, minced
One 14-ounce can crushed tomatoes, preferably San Marzano, including the juices
Kosher or sea salt

1. In a medium skillet, heat 2 tablespoons olive oil over moderate heat. Stir in the garlic and cook until soft, about 2 minutes, being careful not to let the garlic burn. Transfer to a blender.

2. Add the tomatoes and the remaining tablespoon of olive oil to the blender and puree. Add salt to taste, then let cool to room temperature.

PIZZA MARGHERITA WITH TOMATO, MOZZARELLA, AND BASIL

1. Preheat the oven to 500°F. Put the pizza dough on a lightly oiled baking sheet. Using a rolling pin or your fingers, roll out or press the dough into a circle 12 inches in diameter, or press it to the size of the baking sheet, making sure to push it into the corners.

2. Spread the tomato sauce on the dough, leaving a 1-inch border for the crust. Top the sauce with the mozzarella slices.

3. Season with a pinch each of salt and pepper, drizzle with a little olive oil, and sprinkle with the fresh or dried herbs.

4. Bake the pizza for about 9 minutes, until the crust is golden and crispy and the cheese is a little crispy, too. Remove the pizza from the oven, and transfer to a cutting board to cool. Tear the basil leaves into pieces with your hands, and scatter them on top of the pizza. Let the pizza rest for at least 3 minutes before serving.

Basic Pizza Pie Dough (page 149)
½ cup Classic Tomato Sauce
　(page 150) or store-bought pizza
　sauce
1 pound fresh mozzarella, thinly sliced
Salt and freshly ground pepper
Olive oil for drizzling
Leaves from 2 fresh thyme or oregano
　sprigs, or ½ teaspoon dried thyme or
　oregano
20 large fresh basil leaves

PIZZA WITH EGGPLANT, HAM, ARUGULA, AND MOZZARELLA CHEESE

1. Preheat the oven to 500°F. Brush the eggplant rounds generously with oil, and sprinkle lightly with salt and pepper. Cook for 3 to 4 minutes per side in a stovetop grill pan over medium-high heat, or roast in the oven for 8 to 10 minutes, turning the heat down to 425°F while you roast.

2. Put the dough on a lightly oiled baking sheet. Using a rolling pin or your fingers, roll out or press the dough into a circle

One 1-pound eggplant, cut into
　½-inch rounds
Olive oil
Salt and freshly ground pepper
Basic Pizza Pie Dough (page 149)
1 cup Classic Tomato Sauce
　(page 150) or store-bought pizza
　sauce

10 thin slices cured ham, such as
    prosciutto
1½ cups baby arugula or spinach
    leaves
Balsamic vinegar
½ cup shredded fresh mozzarella
    cheese (or freshly grated
    Parmigiano-Reggiano cheese)

12 inches in diameter, or press it to the size of the baking
sheet, making sure to push it into the corners. Spread the tomato sauce on the dough, leaving a 1-inch border for the crust.
Top with the eggplant.

3. Bake the pizza for about 11 minutes, until the edges are
crisp and golden brown. Lay the ham slices on top of the
pizza and bake for 5 minutes longer.

4. Meanwhile, toss the spinach or arugula in a bowl with 2
or 3 tablespoons olive oil, a drizzle of balsamic vinegar, and
salt and pepper to taste. When the pizza has finished cooking, top it with the greens mixture and cheese. Drizzle with a
little more oil and a grind of pepper, if desired. Cut into
wedges and enjoy.

PIZZA WITH BACON, ROSEMARY, AND GOAT CHEESE

Basic Pizza Pie Dough (page 149)
Cornmeal or all-purpose flour, for
    dusting
2 tablespoons olive oil
1 cup Classic Tomato Sauce (page 150),
    or store-bought pizza sauce (optional)
8 ounces soft goat cheese, crumbled
2 tablespoons chopped fresh rosemary
4 ounces thickly sliced bacon, cut into
    1-inch strips, or thinly sliced pancetta
Salt and freshly ground pepper

1. Preheat the oven to 500°F. Place a large rimmed baking
sheet in the oven and heat for 20 to 30 minutes. Meanwhile,
on a lightly floured surface, using a rolling pin or your fingers,
roll out or press the dough to a circle 12 inches in diameter and
brush with 1 tablespoon of oil. Spread the tomato sauce on top
(if using), leaving a 1-inch border for the crust, then sprinkle
with the cheese and top with the rosemary and bacon.

2. Drizzle the remaining tablespoon of oil over the pizza and
season with salt and pepper. Transfer to the heated baking
sheet and bake for about 11 minutes, until the edges are crisp
and golden. Cut into wedges and serve either warm, at room
temperature, or cold.

Marry Me Lasagne

Lasagne with Ricotta Cheese, Mozzarella Cheese, and Basil

Maybe you want to marry him, but aren't an Engagement Chicken kind of girl. Why not ask *him*? Your inspiration: Hillary Seitz, a Los Angeles screenwriter who had been with her boyfriend for seven years when she decided to propose. "He'd wanted to get married all along; I was the one who'd resisted," explained Hillary. "I wanted a proposal that said thanks for hanging in there and having faith in me." So Hillary went to a paint-your-own pottery shop and painted two plates: one with the phrase "Charlie, will you marry me?" and the other with "Please say yes." Hillary took her plates to a favorite restaurant, asked them to serve, and watched as Charlie uncovered the proposal. Naturally, he *did* say yes. Want to try it yourself? Consider this layers-of-love lasagne—big enough, incidentally, to cover the whole plate. Message optional!

Serves 4 to 6

3 cups Marinara Sauce (recipe follows; in a pinch, use your favorite jarred red sauce)

8 ounces uncooked lasagne noodles

One 15- to 16-ounce container whole or part-skim ricotta cheese

3 large eggs

2 cups shredded fresh mozzarella cheese (8 ounces)

½ cup freshly grated Parmigiano-Reggiano cheese

Basil leaves, finely chopped, for garnish

1. Preheat the oven to 350°F. Prepare the marinara sauce. While the sauce is simmering, bring a large pot of salted water to a boil. Drop in the lasagne noodles one at a time and cook over high heat, stirring occasionally, until just al dente, around 5 minutes. Drain the noodles in a colander and set them aside.

2. In a medium bowl, combine the ricotta and eggs. Spread 1 cup marinara sauce in the bottom of a 9- by 13-inch baking dish. Top with a layer of lasagne noodles, followed by half the ricotta mixture.

[CONTINUED]

3. Repeat with a second layer of marinara, noodles, and ricotta mixture and top with a third layer of noodles. Spread ¾ cup marinara sauce on the noodles (reserving ¼ cup to drizzle over each lasagne slice when you serve it). Sprinkle with the mozzarella and Parmigiano-Reggiano cheese.

4. Bake the lasagne for about 1 hour, or until the top is golden, the filling is bubbling around the edges, and the noodles are tender when pierced with a sharp knife. Remove from the oven and let cool for 15 minutes before serving. Cut the lasagne into thick slices, arrange on plates, drizzle with the remaining marinara sauce, and serve, garnished with basil.

MARINARA SAUCE

5 large garlic cloves, thinly sliced

¼ cup olive oil

Two 28-ounce cans whole tomatoes (preferably San Marzano), drained and chopped

Salt and freshly ground black pepper

½ teaspoon red pepper flakes

2 tablespoons unsalted butter

10 basil leaves, torn into pieces

1. In a large saucepan, cook the garlic in the olive oil over moderate heat until golden, about 30 seconds.

2. Turn the heat up to high; add the tomatoes, a large pinch each of salt and pepper, and the red pepper flakes. Bring to a simmer, then turn the heat down to moderately low. Cook, stirring occasionally, until the sauce is thick, 15 to 20 minutes.

3. Add the butter and basil to the saucepan, stirring to melt the butter. Add salt and pepper to taste.

glamour girl tip

This lasagne recipe leaves plenty of room for personalization. Play around with other fillings, adding a layer of sautéed mushrooms, chopped sautéed spinach leaves, or even some cooked crumbled sausage.

We Still Miss
The Sopranos Spaghetti

Spaghetti and Bite-Size Meatballs

Google "spaghetti and meatballs" and more than half a million recipes pop up. Forget all of them and simply commit this one to memory—it's basic enough to make once a week, but the chunky marinara with slivers of garlic and basil give it a fresher, fancier feel. We started making this recipe back in 2002, when *The Sopranos* was still the highlight of our week. Now all we've got are the DVDs—and this killer pasta. Add it to your repertoire and call it your family's secret recipe, passed down for generations. We won't tell Tony.

Serves 2 to 4

MEATBALLS
½ pound ground beef
¼ cup plain bread crumbs
1 large egg, lightly beaten
5 tablespoons grated Parmigiano-
   Reggiano cheese
½ teaspoon minced garlic
½ teaspoon salt
⅛ teaspoon freshly ground pepper
1 tablespoon finely chopped fresh
   flat-leaf parsley
¼ teaspoon dried oregano
1 tablespoon olive oil

MARINARA SAUCE
3 large garlic cloves, thinly sliced
2 tablespoons olive oil
One 28-ounce can whole tomatoes,
   drained and chopped
Salt and freshly ground pepper
1 tablespoon unsalted butter
5 basil leaves, torn into pieces

1. Make the meatballs: In a large bowl, combine all the ingredients except the olive oil, mixing gently with your hands.

2. Rinse your hands with cool water, then lightly shape the meatball mixture into balls the size of a grape.

3. In a large, heavy skillet, heat the olive oil over moderately high heat.

4. Working in batches, arrange the meatballs in the skillet in a single layer and cook, turning a few times, until richly browned on all sides, about 8 minutes total, being careful not to burn them. Transfer to a plate and set aside.

[CONTINUED]

PASTA

One 8-ounce package spaghetti
Freshly grated Parmigiano-Reggiano
  cheese, for serving

5. Make the marinara sauce: In a large saucepan, cook the garlic in the olive oil over moderate heat until golden, about 30 seconds.

6. Turn the heat up to high; add the tomatoes and a large pinch of salt. Bring to a simmer, then turn heat down to moderately low. Cook, stirring occasionally, until the sauce is thick, 15 to 20 minutes.

7. Add the butter and basil to the saucepan, stirring to melt the butter. Add salt and pepper to taste.

8. Add the meatballs to the saucepan, stirring to combine. Simmer until heated through, about 5 minutes longer.

9. Meanwhile, bring a large pot of salted water to a boil. Add the spaghetti and cook according to package instructions until al dente. Drain.

10. Add the spaghetti to the saucepan with the marinara and meatballs and toss to coat. Transfer to a large bowl and serve, passing the cheese at the table.

Let's Make a Baby Pasta

Penne with Spicy Tomato Sauce

We don't know why this pasta is so good at what it does. All we know is that Glamour.com food blogger Sarah Jio has made it three times for her husband; now they have three babies. You do the math.

Serves 2 to 4

Kosher salt

¾ pound penne

2 tablespoons olive oil

2 garlic cloves, minced

½ teaspoon red pepper flakes (or slightly more for spicier results)

One 14-ounce can diced or crushed tomatoes (preferably San Marzano)

¼ cup grated Pecorino Romano or Parmigiano-Reggiano cheese

1. In a large pot, bring water to a boil and add a large pinch of salt.

2. Add the penne to the pot and cook according to package instructions until al dente. Set aside ½ cup of cooking liquid, then drain and reserve the pasta in a serving bowl.

3. Meanwhile, in a large skillet, heat the oil over moderate heat. Add the garlic and red pepper flakes and cook, stirring constantly with a wooden spoon, for about 30 seconds, being careful not to let the garlic brown. Add the tomatoes and crush them with the back of your spoon (leaving the sauce a bit chunky). Simmer until warmed through, about 10 minutes. Add salt to taste. (Sauce will keep for up to three days in the fridge.)

4. Scrape the tomato sauce into the serving bowl with the pasta and toss to coat. Sprinkle the cheese on top and serve— with red wine and candlelight!

I Got Thinner Eating Pasta

Pasta with Fresh Vegetables, Herbs, and Ricotta Cheese

Serves 2 to 4

2 red or yellow bell peppers

One ½-pound eggplant, cut into
    ½-inch pieces

One ½-pound zucchini, cut into
    ½-inch pieces

4 tablespoons extra-virgin olive oil

2 garlic cloves, chopped

6 tablespoons fresh herbs (ideally a
    mix of thyme, sage, and rosemary),
    finely chopped

2 medium red onions, cut into ½-inch
    wedges

2 leeks, pale and green parts only,
    halved lengthwise and cut into
    ¼-inch-thick slices (see tip below on
    cleaning and cutting leeks)

Salt and freshly ground pepper

¾ to 1 pound penne or fusilli (prefer-
    ably whole wheat)

⅓ cup sun-dried tomatoes packed in
    oil, finely chopped

⅓ cup kalamata olives, pitted and
    chopped

If you love carbs like we love carbs, you'll never swear off them entirely. This recipe is the real deal. Our executive editor Lauren Brody once lost 35 pounds of college weight by eating pasta almost every night. She says, "It's all about whole-wheat pasta and portion control." Slow-roasting vegetables with fresh herbs builds layers of low-cal flavor, and the ricotta—part-skim works—makes everything creamy without heavy cheeses. If you haven't tried whole-wheat pasta, don't hesitate: It doesn't work in all dishes, but here it adds an earthy nuttiness that complements the rustic veggies perfectly. Our favorite brands are Barilla Plus, De Cecco, and Bionaturae, all available at supermarkets nationally.

1. Preheat the broiler. Broil the peppers on the top rack 4 to 5 inches from the heat, turning occasionally until the skins are blistered and a little charred, about 9 minutes. Transfer the peppers to a bowl and cover tightly with plastic wrap. Let stand until cool, about 20 minutes. When the peppers are cool enough to handle, peel off the skin, discard the seeds, and chop.

2. Preheat the oven to 400°F. On a large rimmed baking sheet, toss the eggplant and zucchini with 2 tablespoons oil, the garlic, and the chopped herb mixture. Meanwhile, on a second baking sheet, toss the onions and leeks with the

remaining 2 tablespoons oil. Season both with salt and pepper. Spread out in an even layer and roast for 15 to 20 minutes, turning with a spatula a few times, until the vegetables start to brown around the edges. Transfer the vegetables to a bowl and set aside.

3. While the vegetables are roasting, bring a large saucepan of salted water to a boil. Add the pasta and cook according to package instructions until al dente. Drain.

4. Add the pasta to the bowl with the roasted vegetables. Add the sun-dried tomatoes, olives, basil, parsley, Parmigiano-Reggiano, and salt and pepper to taste. Toss well to combine. Serve with the ricotta in a small bowl on the side for stirring into pasta.

⅓ cup chopped fresh basil

⅓ cup chopped fresh flat-leaf parsley

½ cup freshly grated Parmigiano-Reggiano cheese

1 cup whole milk or part-skim ricotta cheese, for serving

glamour girl tip

Leeks need to be cleaned thoroughly before cooking. First, trim them just above the roots, then cut away the dark green leaves from the other end of the stalk. With a small sharp knife, cut the leek from end to end, halfway through to the center core. Pull back the leaves and flush out all the dirt under running water. Shake to dry before following any other cooking instructions.

Instant Happiness Mac and Cheese

Macaroni with Four Cheeses and Crumb Topping

Serves 4

TOPPING

1 tablespoon unsalted butter, melted

¼ cup bread crumbs (preferably panko, the Japanese variety now available in many supermarkets)

2 tablespoons freshly grated Parmigiano-Reggiano cheese

MACARONI

½ pound elbow macaroni (half the box)

2 tablespoons unsalted butter, plus more for greasing the baking dish

1½ tablespoons all-purpose flour

1 cup whole milk

1 cup coarsely grated extra-sharp Cheddar cheese (about 4 ounces)

1 cup coarsely grated fontina cheese (about 4 ounces)

1 cup coarsely grated Gruyère cheese (about 4 ounces)

2 tablespoons freshly grated Parmigiano-Reggiano cheese

Salt and freshly ground pepper

This macaroni and cheese magically brokers a truce between children's cravings for a creamy, classic dish and the adult desire for something more sophisticated than bright yellow box fare. *Everyone* loves this version. The trick is using four cheeses: Cheddar + fontina + Gruyère + Parmigiano-Reggiano = luxury on a plate.

1. Preheat the oven to 400°F and position the oven rack in the middle of the oven.

2. Make the topping: In a small bowl, combine the melted butter with the bread crumbs and Parmigiano-Reggiano cheese, stirring well. Set aside.

3. Make the macaroni: Butter a 1- to 1½-quart glass or ceramic baking dish or a 9-inch pie dish and set it aside. Bring a large pot of salted water to a boil. Add the macaroni and cook according to package directions, until al dente. Reserve ¼ cup cooking water and drain the macaroni in a colander.

4. Make the cheese sauce: In a small heavy saucepan, melt the 2 tablespoons butter over moderately low heat and whisk in the flour until smooth. Cook the mixture (called a roux), whisking constantly, for 1 minute, then whisk in the milk. Turn the heat up to high and bring the sauce to a boil, whisk-

ing constantly. Turn the heat down to low and simmer, whisking occasionally, for 2 minutes longer. Add the cheeses, whisking, until melted and smooth. Add salt and pepper to taste.

5. In a large bowl, combine the macaroni, reserved cooking water, and cheese sauce, stirring to coat. Transfer to the prepared baking dish. Sprinkle the bread crumb topping evenly over the macaroni and bake 20 minutes, until golden and bubbling. Let rest 5 minutes before serving.

VARIATION 1: SPICY MEXICAN MAC AND CHEESE

Prepare as above, but use shredded Monterey Jack or pepper Jack cheese instead of the four-cheese blend, and stir cayenne, ground cumin, dried oregano, and chili powder—and, if desired, chicken—into the cheese sauce. Omit the bread crumb topping and use finely crushed tortilla chips as the topping instead.

3 cups shredded Monterey Jack or pepper Jack cheese

⅛ teaspoon cayenne

2 teaspoons ground cumin

½ teaspoon dried oregano

2 teaspoons chili powder

2 cups shredded cooked chicken (optional)

Tortilla chips, finely crushed

VARIATION 2: ITALIAN MAC AND CHEESE

Prepare as above, but instead of the four-cheese blend, use mozzarella or fontina cheese and freshly grated Parmigiano-Reggiano. Stir tomatoes into the cheese sauce, and omit the reserved pasta cooking water.

[CONTINUED]

2½ cups shredded mozzarella or fontina cheese

½ cup freshly grated Parmigiano-Reggiano cheese

1 14-ounce can stewed tomatoes, drained and finely chopped

VARIATION 3: MIXED MUSHROOM MAC AND CHEESE

2 shallots, finely chopped

1 pound mixed mushrooms, thinly sliced

2 tablespoons butter

2 tablespoons olive oil

3 cups Gruyère cheese

Prepare as above, but sauté shallots and mushrooms in butter and olive oil over moderate heat, until softened. Instead of the four-cheese blend, use Gruyère cheese, and stir the mushroom mixture into the cheese sauce.

glamour girl tip

Buy solid cheeses and blend them all—minus the Parmigiano-Reggiano—together in a food processor. If the grocery doesn't have fontina or Gruyère, replace with any other semisoft or hard white cheeses, taking care to avoid feta and blue cheese.

Happy Mess Pasta with Chorizo and Clams

Linguine with Littlenecks, Spicy Sausage, and Toasted Bread

One of our editors loves colorful, sloppy pastas—and used to eat them frequently for lunch. Then one day, she went to pick up her dry cleaning and the owner said, "My dear, it's not that I don't love your business. But you dress like a woman and eat like a child." It took the bluntness—and kindness—of a stranger for her to realize that as much as she loves linguine, she cannot have it for lunch. Now she goes home at night, changes into a T-shirt and jeans, and whips up this dish—absolutely scrumptious and perfect for casual, sexy evenings when you don't mind making a little mess.

Serves 4

1 pound linguine

2 tablespoons olive oil

1 garlic clove, minced

4 ounces Mexican chorizo (uncooked) or other spicy pork sausage, casing removed

1 link Spanish chorizo (precooked) or about 4 ounces pepperoni, casing removed and meat chopped

One 28-ounce can crushed tomatoes, preferably San Marzano

2 pounds littleneck clams, rinsed and scrubbed in cold water to remove the grit

Salt and freshly ground pepper

4 thick slices crusty bread, toasted, for serving

1. Bring a large saucepan of salted water to a boil. Add the linguine and cook according to package instructions until al dente. Drain in a colander and set aside.

2. Meanwhile, in a large, heavy-bottomed pot, heat the oil over moderate heat. Add the garlic and cook, stirring, until golden, about 30 seconds. Add the sausage and cook, breaking up any lumps with a spoon, about 2 minutes.

3. Add the tomatoes to the pot. Turn the heat down to low and simmer, stirring occasionally, until the sauce is thick, 12 to 15 minutes. Meanwhile, scrub any remaining sand off the clamshells, discarding any that are already open.

[CONTINUED]

4. Add the clams to the pot. Increase the heat to moderately high and cover. Cook about 10 minutes, stirring a few times, until all the clams have opened (discard any that remain closed). Add salt and pepper to the sauce as needed.

5. Arrange the linguine in bowls. Top with the chorizo-clam sauce and serve with toasted bread on the side.

kitchen basics:
Thirty-Minute Pasta Recipes and Sauces

This chart—a *Glamour* classic first published in our working-woman cookbook *Gourmet on the Run*—makes pasta dinners perfectly simple. Once you get the rhythm, you'll feel comfortable experimenting with your own favorite add-ins. Each recipe serves four.

Tomato-based technique. Heat 2 tablespoons olive oil over medium heat in a large skillet. Add the flavor makers (for your choice of sauce) and cook over moderately high heat, about 1 minute. Add 1 28-ounce can chopped peeled tomatoes. Simmer over medium-low heat 15 minutes more. Meanwhile, prepare 1 pound of pasta according to package instructions (see pasta tips, page 168, for ideas on which shape to choose). In the skillet, add the finishing touches for your chosen sauce. Simmer 5 minutes. Toss the sauce with the cooked pasta and add salt and pepper to taste. Add the garnish that goes with your sauce.

Cream-based technique. In a large skillet, cook the flavor makers over moderately high heat for 5 to 8 minutes. Add the finishing touches for your chosen sauce; heat through for another 3 to 4 minutes. Meanwhile, prepare the pasta according to package directions. Toss the pasta with the sauce and garnish that goes with it.

TOMATO-BASED	FLAVOR MAKERS	FINISHING TOUCHES	GARNISHES
Amatriciana	1 garlic clove, crushed; ¼ teaspoon red pepper flakes; one 2-ounce can anchovies, drained and chopped (optional)	4 ounces bacon or pancetta, cooked and crumbled	2 tablespoons chopped fresh flat-leaf parsley
Puttanesca	2 garlic cloves, crushed; ¼ teaspoon red pepper flakes; one 2-ounce can anchovies, drained	¼ cup oil-cured olives, drained and pitted	2 tablespoons chopped fresh flat-leaf parsley; 2 tablespoons capers, rinsed
Zucchini-Eggplant	2 garlic cloves, crushed; 1 pound eggplant, cut into ½-inch cubes	2 cups sliced zucchini; 1 roasted red pepper, chopped	2 tablespoons chopped basil
CREAM-BASED	**FLAVOR MAKERS**	**FINISHING TOUCHES**	**GARNISHES**
Carbonara*	8 ounces bacon, diced	⅓ cup half-and-half; ½ teaspoon freshly ground black pepper	¾ cup freshly grated Parmigiano-Reggiano cheese; 3 raw eggs, beaten (see Note below); 2 tablespoons chopped fresh flat-leaf parsley
Romana	1 tablespoon butter; ½ cup chopped ham or prosciutto; 3 cups sliced mushrooms (8 ounces)	1¼ cups half-and-half; 1½ cups cooked green peas	½ cup freshly grated Parmigiano-Reggiano cheese
Walnut-Basil	1 tablespoon butter; 2 garlic cloves, minced; 2 cups chopped fresh basil	1¼ cups half-and-half; 1 cup chopped toasted walnuts	¾ cup freshly grated Parmigiano-Reggiano cheese

*NOTE: Adding the raw eggs to the pasta while it's still hot is the classic way of making pasta carbonara, but pregnant women and those with compromised immune systems should check with their physician first. To be safe, make sure to use fresh eggs, and don't let the dish sit out for too long. The carbonara recipe can also be made without eggs.

Which Pastas Go with Which Sauces?

Ever wonder what's up with all the different pasta shapes out there, and why some recipes call for fusilli while others ask for spaghetti or linguine? Choosing which type of pasta to use with which sauce is not an exact science—but it's not totally random, either.

Curly Pastas. Some pastas, like fusilli, scoop up sauce in their crevices, so they will work well with chunkier sauces made with meat or vegetables (see our Pasta with Fresh Vegetables, Herbs, and Ricotta Cheese, page 158).

Tube-Shaped Pastas. Pastas such as penne or rigatoni bring assertive texture to a dish and complement a wide range of sauces—they'll stand up to spicy arrabbiata (page 157) or a hearty meat sauce, or add personality to a simple one of olive oil, sautéed garlic, and freshly grated Parmigiano-Reggiano cheese.

Small Pastas. Tiny ones with pretty shapes like shells or orrecchiette (ears), make a nice addition to soups.

The Classic. Spaghetti is one of the most versatile pastas, and it's a time-honored choice for marinara sauce with meatballs.

meat-free mains

Engagement Paella

Paella with Smoked Tofu and Chorizo-Style Veggie Sausages

If you or your guy don't eat meat, Engagement Chicken is not the dish for you. *This* is. Paella offers the same impressive display of home cooking, but with a Latin flair and an all-vegetarian ingredient list. The play of flavors and colors here—yellow rice, green peas, red peppers, smoked tofu—is so enticing that even meat lovers find it impossible to resist. Put the pan on the table and serve straight from it like they do in Spain.

Serves 6

5 cups vegetable broth
1 tablespoon tomato paste
2 teaspoons sweet paprika
½ teaspoon turmeric
2 teaspoons salt
¼ cup olive oil
8 ounces smoked tofu
Four 6- to 7-ounce chorizo-style
    vegetarian protein sausages
1 medium onion, chopped
5 garlic cloves, finely chopped
½ red bell pepper, seeded and thinly
    sliced
½ green bell pepper, seeded and
    thinly sliced
1½ cups medium-grain (or bomba) rice
1 cup grape tomatoes, halved lengthwise
One 9-ounce package frozen
    artichokes, thawed and quartered
    lengthwise
½ cup frozen peas, thawed
2 tablespoons chopped fresh flat-leaf
    parsley
1 lemon

1. In a medium saucepan, bring 3 cups vegetable broth, tomato paste, paprika, turmeric, and salt to a boil, then turn the heat down low to a bare simmer, keeping the saucepan partially covered.

2. Heat the olive oil in a 12-inch-deep heavy nonstick or cast-iron skillet over moderate heat. Add and cook the whole block of tofu and sausages, turning once, until browned all over, about 3 minutes. Transfer to a cutting board, then cut them into ½-inch pieces and reserve.

3. Add the onion, garlic, and peppers to the skillet and cook, stirring occasionally, until the vegetables begin to soften, about 3 minutes. Add the rice to the vegetables and cook, stirring, until the rice is well coated with the oil, about 2 minutes.

[CONTINUED]

4. Add the tofu, sausage, tomatoes, artichokes, and 3 cups of the simmering vegetable stock. Stir well to distribute the ingredients evenly. Turn the heat down to low and cook without stirring, until most of the liquid is absorbed, 6 to 8 minutes. Add the remaining 2 cups vegetable broth and scatter the peas over the surface of the rice. Continue cooking, without stirring, until the liquid is absorbed and the rice is al dente, 8 to 10 minutes longer. Sprinkle with parsley and serve with lemon wedges.

Who Calls a Meeting at 5:00 P.M.? Stir-Fry

Flash-Sautéed Vegetables with Peanuts and Sesame-Soy Sauce

As the person who brings the words and art together on every page of *Glamour*, production director Mari Gill works strenuous hours, often arriving home long past dinner. This easy veggie stir-fry is her late-night staple; the trick is buying precut veggies to eliminate prep work. Next time *you're* stuck at the office (gee, thanks for the end-of-day two-hour powwow, boss!), close your eyes and know that you won't go hungry tonight.

Serves 4

RICE (OPTIONAL)

1 to 2 cups rice

SAUCE

5 tablespoons soy sauce

2 tablespoons red wine vinegar

2 teaspoons sesame oil

¼ cup rice wine (optional)

1 tablespoon grated fresh ginger

1 tablespoon sugar (optional)

STIR-FRY

1 cup broccoli florets, chopped

1 cup cauliflower florets, chopped

½ cup carrots, peeled and chopped

1 tablespoon olive oil

½ onion, cut into thick slices

½ red or green bell pepper, cut into
1-inch slices

1 cup snow peas or sugar snap peas

1 garlic clove, minced

½ cup chopped peanuts or sliced
drained water chestnuts

1. If cooking the rice, begin to cook according to package instructions.

2. Meanwhile, make the sauce: In a medium bowl, whisk all the ingredients together, whisking to dissolve the sugar (if using). Set aside.

3. Make the stir-fry: In a wok or very large skillet over high heat, bring 1 cup water to a boil. Add the broccoli, cauliflower, and carrots, and cover. Cook for 5 minutes. Using a slotted spoon, transfer the vegetables to a large bowl and set aside. Wipe out the wok to eliminate all of the moisture.

4. Add the oil to the wok or skillet and heat over high heat. Add the onion, bell pepper, and peas and cook, stirring, for 3 to 4 minutes, or until the onion is browned.

[CONTINUED]

5. Add the garlic, broccoli, cauliflower, and carrots to the mixture, along with the peanuts or water chestnuts. Cook 1 to 2 minutes, stirring frequently, until warmed through.

6. Add the stir-fry sauce to the wok and stir to coat. Cook an additional 1 to 2 minutes, stirring frequently. Serve over rice, if desired.

Meatless Monday Portobello Burgers

Broiled Mushroom, Red Onion, and Arugula Sandwiches on Country Bread

Inspired by Stella McCartney's Meat Free Monday campaign—designed to encourage one vegetarian day a week, a small change with massive environmental benefits—we created this yummy burger. You won't miss the beef. The dish is he-man satisfying as is.

Serves 4

1 garlic clove
2 ounces roasted red pepper from a jar, drained
½ cup mayonnaise
1 tablespoon Dijon mustard
1 tablespoon fresh lemon juice
Scant ¼ teaspoon cayenne
½ cup freshly grated Parmigiano-Reggiano cheese
½ cup extra-virgin olive oil, plus more for brushing
Four 4-inch-diameter portobello mushrooms, stems removed
Four ¼-inch-thick slices red onion
½ teaspoon salt
¼ teaspoon pepper
8 thick slices good Italian country bread, large enough to hold the mushrooms
2 loosely packed cups baby arugula

1. In a food processor or blender, puree the garlic, red pepper, mayonnaise, mustard, lemon juice, cayenne, and Parmigiano-Reggiano until smooth. With the motor running, add ¼ cup of olive oil in a thin stream until blended and slightly thickened. Set aside.

2. Preheat the broiler. Line a large rimmed baking sheet with foil. Arrange the mushrooms top sides up on the baking sheet side by side with the onion slices. Brush the tops of the mushrooms and onion slices with olive oil and season with the salt and pepper. Broil the mushrooms and onion slices about 3 inches from the heat for about 10 minutes, until tender and lightly charred in spots.

[CONTINUED]

3. Lightly brush the bread slices on one side only with the remaining ¼ cup olive oil, then broil, without turning, about 1 minute, until lightly golden on the oiled sides.

4. Arrange the bread slices on a work surface, toasted side up. Top 4 slices with 1 portobello mushroom, 1 onion slice, and ½ cup arugula leaves each. Spread the roasted red pepper sauce on the remaining 4 slices, close the burgers, and serve.

Let's Eat with Our Fingers Quesadillas

Sweet Onion, Potato, and Goat Cheese Quesadillas

Glamour contributing editor Jessica Strul considers herself generally kitchen averse. No matter—she still wows crowds with this simple finger-food favorite. "It's as easy as salting the rim of your margarita glass," she says, "which I also recommend." (For that handy trick, see page 67.)

Serves 2

2 tablespoons olive oil, plus more for brushing

1 large sweet onion, such as Vidalia or Walla Walla, thinly sliced

1 large russet baking potato, peeled and diced

½ cup water

¼ teaspoon salt

¼ teaspoon pepper

3 ounces mild goat cheese, crumbled, or ¾ cup shredded Monterey Jack cheese

½ cup chopped fresh cilantro

Four 6- to 7-inch flour tortillas

Sour cream, for serving

1. In a large heavy skillet, heat the oil over moderately high heat. Add the onion and cook, stirring often, until golden, about 6 minutes. Turn the heat down to low and stir in the potato, water, salt, and pepper, and simmer, covered, until the potato is soft, about 8 minutes. Transfer to a bowl and stir in the goat cheese and cilantro.

2. Arrange the tortillas on a work surface. Spread the lower halves with the onion mixture, then fold the top halves over to form half-moons. Lightly brush both sides with olive oil.

3. Lightly oil a grill pan or heavy skillet and heat over moderately high heat. Working in two batches, add 2 quesadillas and cook, turning once, until the cheese is melted and the tortilla is golden, about 2 minutes per side. Transfer to a cutting board and cut in half. Repeat with the remaining quesadillas. Serve with sour cream on the side.

[CONTINUED]

2 sweet red bell peppers, chopped

2 garlic cloves, minced

¾ cup shredded pepper Jack cheese

Sauté the onion with the bell peppers, garlic, salt, and pepper. Omit the potato and water. Instead of the goat cheese, use shredded Monterey Jack cheese. Stir in the cilantro, and continue to follow the remaining instructions for the quesadilla recipe.

VARIATION 2: BLACK BEAN AND CORN QUESADILLAS

1 cup frozen corn

½ cup canned black beans, drained

¾ cup shredded cheese (a blend of Jack and Cheddar is ideal)

Sauté the onion, then add frozen corn and black beans. Cook until just heated through. Omit the water and potato. Stir in the salt and pepper, transfer the mixture to a bowl, and stir in shredded cheese along with the cilantro. Follow the remaining instructions for the quesadilla recipe.

glamour girl tip

For best results, look for flour tortillas *not* labeled "fat-free." In our opinion, the few calories you save are just not worth the sacrifice in taste.

I'm Really Stuffed Peppers

Bell Peppers with Couscous, Feta Cheese, and Pine Nuts

Who says you need meat to make it a real meal? This recipe originally appeared in *Glamour* under the headline "Veggie Mains That Satisfy Like Steak," and it does.

1. Bring a large pot of water to a boil. Slice the tops off the peppers; clean out the seeds and veins. Add the tops and bottoms to the pot and boil over high heat for 7 to 10 minutes, or until just tender (not mushy!). Drain (or gently remove from the water with tongs) and immediately plunge into a large bowl of ice water to stop the cooking.

2. In a small skillet, toast the pine nuts over moderate heat for about 6 minutes, until golden brown. Shake the pan while toasting, to avoid burning the pine nuts. Transfer to a plate and let cool.

3. Cook the couscous according to package instructions. Transfer the couscous to a bowl and toss with the toasted pine nuts, herbs, feta cheese, and chickpeas. Add 1 to 2 tablespoons olive oil, lemon juice, and salt and pepper to taste.

4. Fill the peppers with the couscous mixture. Serve.

Serves 4

4 to 6 large red or yellow bell peppers
¼ cup pine nuts
One 6-ounce package couscous
¼ to ½ cup chopped fresh herbs (any combination of basil, dill, mint, or flat-leaf parsley)
½ cup crumbled feta cheese
1 can chickpeas, drained
Olive oil
Juice of 1 lemon
Salt and freshly ground pepper

Pride and Prejudice Shepherd's Pie

Roasted Vegetable Casserole with Creamy Mashed Potato Topping

Serves 4 to 6

4 small red potatoes, peeled and
   chopped (about 3 cups)

Salt

¾ cup milk

2 tablespoons butter

1 cup fresh or frozen thawed peas

Freshly ground pepper

4 tablespoons olive oil

5 garlic cloves, minced

1 medium onion, minced

2 plum tomatoes, chopped

1 cup vegetable broth

2 cups white button mushrooms,
   halved

2 cups chopped leeks, thoroughly
   cleaned of any grit

2 cups chopped zucchini or chopped
   red, yellow, or green bell peppers

1 cup diced peeled parsnips or carrots

2 tablespoons curry powder

1 teaspoon ground cumin

1 tablespoon minced fresh flat-leaf
   parsley

If you love any film in which the heroine spends most of the movie dressed in a corset—or if you read Jane Austen like other women read *Twilight*—then this dinner's right up your nineteenth-century alley. Traditional English shepherd's pie, though, is made with lamb and tends to be quite heavy; we've kept the crispy potato top and created a lighter filling of curry-infused vegetables. It's the perfect dish for a wintry Saturday night in.

1. In a large saucepan, cover the potatoes with cold water and add a large pinch of salt. Bring to a boil and cook over high heat until fork-tender, about 5 minutes. Drain in a colander and return to the saucepan. Using a potato masher or large fork, smash the potatoes to a coarse puree. While they're still very hot, gently stir in the milk, butter, peas, and salt and pepper to taste. Set aside.

2. Preheat the oven to 400°F. Heat 3 tablespoons olive oil in a large saucepan over moderate heat. Add the garlic and cook, stirring constantly with a wooden spoon to avoid burning, until softened, 1 minute. Add the onion and cook until softened, about 5 minutes. Add the tomatoes and cook, stirring constantly, about 2 minutes longer.

3. Add the broth, vegetables, curry powder, and cumin, and bring to a boil. Cover and cook over low heat until the vegetables have softened, between 5 and 10 minutes. Add salt and pepper to taste.

4. Coat the bottom of an 8-by-8-inch baking dish with the remaining tablespoon of olive oil. Using a slotted spoon, transfer the cooked vegetables to the dish. Cover the vegetables with a layer of the mashed potatoes, forming a few small peaks here and there with the back of a spoon.

5. Bake for about 25 minutes, until the top is golden and the filling is bubbling. Some of the mashed potato peaks should be slightly browned and crunchy. Let the pie rest 5 minutes before serving. Sprinkle the top with minced parsley and serve.

glamour girl tip

Leeks need to be cleaned thoroughly before cooking. First, trim them just above the roots, then cut away the dark green leaves from the other end of the stalk. With a small sharp knife, cut the leek from end to end, halfway through to the center core. Pull back the leaves and flush out all the dirt under running water. Shake to dry before following any other cooking instructions.

I'm So Here for You Eggplant Parmesan

Layered Eggplant with Tomato-Basil Sauce and Melted Mozzarella Cheese

Serves 6 to 8

2½ pounds eggplant (about 3 medium), cut crosswise into ⅓-inch-thick rounds

4 teaspoons salt

Two 28-ounce cans whole tomatoes, including their juices

1½ cups plus 3 tablespoons olive oil

1 medium onion, finely chopped

2 large garlic cloves, finely chopped

5 fresh basil leaves, coarsely chopped

1⅓ cups all-purpose flour

¼ teaspoon black pepper

¾ cup freshly grated Parmigiano-Reggiano cheese

6 large eggs

1½ cups bread crumbs

1 pound fresh mozzarella cheese, thinly sliced

This recipe is a fairly large undertaking—there are a lot of steps, and frying the eggplant will take at least twenty minutes—but it is truly worth it. Like Marry Me Lasagne (page 153), it telegraphs comfort—but it involves no pasta, and the layers of crispy eggplant make it especially hearty. It's the perfect dish to bring to a friend going through anything stressful (bonus points if she's a new mom!). Carry it over cold and she can warm it in a 350°F oven (stick a Post-it on top with the instructions so she won't have to call you if she forgets). It also freezes nicely for future comfort eating.

1. Preheat the oven to 375°F and position an oven rack in the middle of the oven. In a colander set over a bowl, toss the eggplant with 2 teaspoons salt, then let drain 30 minutes. Rinse and pat dry. (Don't skip this step: It keeps your parm from being watery!)

2. Meanwhile, in a blender, working in batches, coarsely puree the tomatoes and their juices. In a 5-quart heavy pot, heat 3 tablespoons olive oil over moderately high heat. Add the onion and garlic and cook, stirring, until softened, about 6 minutes. Add the tomato puree, basil, and 1 teaspoon salt. Turn the heat down to low and simmer, uncovered, stirring occasionally, until slightly thickened, 25 to 30 minutes. Set aside.

3. In a shallow bowl, stir together the flour, ½ teaspoon salt, ¼ teaspoon pepper, and ⅓ cup Parmigiano-Reggiano cheese. In a second shallow bowl, lightly whisk the eggs with ¼ cup water and the remaining ½ teaspoon salt. In a third shallow bowl, spread the bread crumbs.

4. Working with 1 eggplant slice at a time, dredge the eggplant in the flour mixture, shaking off the excess. Dip the slice in the egg mixture, letting the excess drip off. Dredge in the bread crumbs until evenly coated. Transfer the coated eggplant slices to sheets of wax paper.

5. Heat the remaining 1½ cups oil in a 12-inch-deep non-stick skillet over moderately high heat until hot but not smoking, then fry the eggplant 4 slices at a time, until golden brown, turning over once, 5 to 6 minutes per batch. Transfer with tongs to paper towels to drain.

6. Lightly oil a 3- to 3½-quart glass or ceramic dish. Spread 1½ cups of the reserved tomato sauce in the bottom of the baking dish. Arrange about one third of the eggplant slices in a single layer over the sauce, overlapping slightly if necessary. Cover the eggplant with about one third of the remaining sauce, one third of the Parmigiano-Reggiano cheese, and one third of the mozzarella. Continue layering with the remaining eggplant, sauce, Parmigiano-Reggiano, and mozzarella, ending with a layer of mozzarella.

7. Tightly cover the baking dish with a sheet of oiled foil. Bake for about 20 minutes, until the cheese is melted. Uncover and bake until the cheese is golden and the sauce is bubbling, about 25 minutes longer. Let stand 15 minutes before serving.

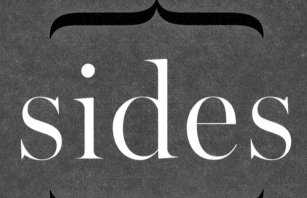

I'll Take Care of You Mashed Potatoes

Creamy, Old-Fashioned Mashed Potatoes

These potatoes are a perfect example of how less is often more with cooking. Some milk, a pinch of nutmeg and a little (okay, *a lot of*) butter is all you need to make these the most delicious—and therefore most comforting—mashies you've ever tasted.

Use any kind of potatoes you want; the trick is mixing the ingredients while the potatoes are still super hot, so that the flavors blend seamlessly. And if you salt the potato water generously, you shouldn't have to add any salt after mashing.

Serves 4

2 pounds potatoes, peeled and cut
   into 2-inch pieces
Salt
1 cup milk
6 to 8 tablespoons butter
Pinch of freshly ground nutmeg
Freshly ground pepper

1. In a large saucepan, cover the potatoes with cold water and add a large pinch of salt. Bring to a boil and cook over high heat until tender when pierced with a fork, about 25 minutes.

2. Drain the potatoes and return them to the saucepan. Using a potato masher or a large serving fork, coarsely mash.

3. While the potatoes are still very hot, stir in the milk and butter. Add nutmeg, salt, and pepper to taste. Serve.

glamour girl tip

It's always better to hand-mash potatoes using a masher or even a large fork so that you don't overwork them (overbeating—easy to do with an electric mixer or food processor—breaks down the cells and releases starch, resulting in gummy, pasty potatoes).

Easy Peasy Risi e Bisi

Italian-Style Rice and Peas with Tangy Parmesan Cheese

Serves 2 as a main course or
4 as an appetizer

1 tablespoon olive oil

1 small onion, chopped

3 garlic cloves, chopped

½ cup orzo

1¼ cups chicken or vegetable stock or
   low-sodium broth

¾ cup water

Salt and freshly ground pepper

⅓ cup freshly grated Parmigiano-
   Reggiano cheese

1 cup frozen peas

Risi e bisi is Italian slang for "rice and peas." Our version is easy to pull off, since we use frozen peas and orzo (a ricelike pasta that cooks up risotto soft without risotto effort). The dish is so rich and creamy, it's good enough to eat as an entrée—but so simple you can whip it up as a side dish for fish or meat. (It's also fun to say in a fake Italian accent: *rrrrrrrrrisi e bisi!*)

1. In a small saucepan, heat the oil over moderate heat. Add the onion and garlic and cook, stirring a few times, until golden and softened, about 6 minutes.

2. Add the orzo to the saucepan and cook, stirring, for 2 minutes.

3. Add the stock and water and season to taste with salt and pepper. If using low-sodium broth, season more generously.

4. Bring the stock to a boil, then turn the heat down to low and simmer, covered, for 20 minutes, stirring occasionally, until the orzo is tender.

5. Stir in the cheese and peas (feel free to add more than just 1 cup of peas; some people prefer more). Add more salt and pepper to taste. Cook for 5 more minutes, until the cheese has melted and the peas are warmed through. Serve.

Best Supporting Side Dish Cabernet Mushrooms

Mushrooms Sautéed with Garlic and Red Onion

Serving mushrooms and onions with steak is nothing new, but these wine-infused 'shrooms take the classic pairing to the next level. Using fancier varieties like shiitake, oyster, and portobello gives the dish a robust, earthy flavor that won't get lost on the plate. And caramelizing the onions—a sugar-releasing process that happens when you sauté them over high heat—adds a needed touch of sweetness. Drink the leftover cabernet with dinner (as if we had to tell you that).

Serves 2

3 tablespoons olive oil

2 garlic cloves, minced

1 small or medium red onion, sliced into thin half-moon slices

2 cups quartered mushrooms (preferably shiitake, oyster, or baby portobellos)

½ cup dry red wine, such as cabernet sauvignon

1 tablespoon minced fresh flat-leaf parsley

Kosher salt and ground pepper

1. In a medium skillet, heat the olive oil over moderately high heat.

2. Add the garlic and onions and cook, stirring, for 2 minutes. Turn the heat up to high and add the mushrooms. Cook, stirring often, until they begin to soften, about 4 minutes. Pour in the wine and bring to a boil. Turn the heat down to low and simmer for about 10 minutes, stirring occasionally, until the mushrooms are softened and the sauce is thickened.

3. Sprinkle the mushrooms with parsley, and season to taste with salt and pepper. Serve immediately.

Beyond Basic Broccoli

Broccoli with Garlic, Olive Oil, and Sea Salt

Serves 2 to 4

One 1½-pound head broccoli, bottom
   2 inches trimmed off, broccoli cut
   into florets
3 tablespoons extra-virgin olive oil
4 garlic cloves, thinly sliced
Sea salt and freshly ground black
   pepper
½ teaspoon crushed red pepper flakes
   (optional)

Adding a little garlic and a few red pepper flakes to your florets will have everyone at the table asking for your secret. Crunchy, bright, with just a kiss of heat, this dish is the perfect thing to serve with chicken, fish, or steak; toss the cold leftovers into a salad.

1. Bring a medium pot of salted water to a boil. Meanwhile, fill a large bowl with ice water. Add broccoli to the boiling water and cook, uncovered, until tender when pierced with a fork, about 5 minutes. Using tongs, immediately transfer the broccoli to the ice water, then drain in a colander. Wipe out the pot.

2. Add the olive oil and garlic to the pot and cook over moderately high heat, stirring occasionally, until just golden, 1 minute. Add the broccoli and cook, stirring frequently, until heated through, 2 minutes. Add salt and pepper to taste, and crushed red pepper flakes (if using).

Just Kiss Me Garlic Bread

Buttery Garlic Loaf

Look, garlic is garlic. It's got serious, tongue-tingling flavor—but as long as you're *both* eating it, what's wrong with that? In this classic *Glamour* recipe, cutting slits in the bread helps the buttery goodness soak all the way through. A perfect side for lasagne (page 153) or spaghetti and meatballs (page 155), this garlic bread also goes nicely with a salad or soup.

Serves 6

4 garlic cloves, peeled
½ cup unsalted butter, softened
1½ tablespoons chopped fresh
   flat-leaf parsley
Salt and freshly ground pepper
1 French baguette or Italian loaf

1. Preheat the oven to 350°F. Using a garlic press, a mortar and pestle, or the back of a large, heavy knife, crush the garlic cloves. In a small bowl, combine the butter, garlic, and parsley and mix well. Season to taste with salt and pepper.

2. Make shallow cuts in the bread loaf at approximately 2-inch intervals as if you're making slices, but be sure not to cut all the way down to the bottom. Push 1 teaspoon of the butter mixture into each slice. (Alternatively, slice the loaf of bread in half lengthwise and spread the butter mixture on each side.) Dab any extra garlic-butter mix on the outside of the loaf.

3. Wrap the loaf completely in aluminum foil and transfer it to the oven. Bake for 15 to 20 minutes, until the bread is crisp and the garlic is fragrant. Slice and serve.

kitchen basics:

Five Irresistible Vegetable Side Dishes

Whether you're already a veggie fanatic or still not convinced that you love them, here are a few more deliciously simple, nutrient-packed recipes that will help you fall hard.

ROASTED BUTTERNUT SQUASH

Serves 2 to 3

1 large butternut squash
4 garlic cloves, minced
2 tablespoons diced butter
3 tablespoons olive oil
2 tablespoons maple syrup
Salt and freshly ground
  black pepper

1. Preheat the oven to 400°F, then peel the squash, scrape out the seeds, and cut the flesh into 1-inch cubes.

2. Put the squash on a large rimmed baking sheet, sprinkle with minced garlic and diced butter, and drizzle with olive oil and maple syrup. Toss all the ingredients together well, season with 1 teaspoon salt and ½ teaspoon pepper, and roast for 20 minutes.

3. Using a spatula or tongs, turn the squash over, then roast for about 20 minutes longer, until softened and nicely browned. Transfer to a platter and serve.

BUTTER-AND-HERB-ROASTED ONIONS

Serves 6

6 medium red onions
1 stick butter (½ cup)

1. Position a rack in the center of the oven; preheat the oven to 400°F. Peel onions and cut each vertically into 6 wedges within ½ inch of the bottom (don't cut all the way through). Place the onions on a

rimmed baking sheet. Open the onion wedges to resemble flowers but do not break the wedges off the base. Set aside.

2. In a small saucepan, melt butter over low heat. Whisk in rosemary, parsley, and lemon juice. Add salt and pepper to taste, then brush some of the herb butter over the onions.

3. Transfer the onions to the oven and roast until tender and beginning to char, brushing occasionally with more herb butter, about 1 hour. Serve warm.

4 teaspoons minced fresh rosemary
1 tablespoon chopped fresh flat-leaf parsley
2 teaspoons fresh lemon juice
Salt and freshly ground pepper

SWEET POTATO FRIES WITH CRISPY SAGE

1. In a 4-inch-deep heavy pot or deep fryer fitted with a thermometer, heat 2 inches of vegetable oil to 360°F. (If you don't have a thermometer, drop a kernel of popcorn into the oil; the kernel will pop when the oil is hot enough—in the 350°F to 365°F range.)

2. Preheat the oven to 200°F. Peel sweet potatoes and cut them into sticks about ½-inch thick. Put flour in a large resealable plastic bag, then add the sweet potatoes. Seal the bag with lots of air and toss to coat the sweet potatoes.

3. Working in small batches, shake off any excess flour and carefully add the sweet potatoes to the hot oil. Fry, stirring occasionally, until golden and tender, about 5 minutes. Using a slotted spoon, transfer the sweet potatoes to paper towels to drain. Sprinkle with salt.

Serves 4

Vegetable oil
3 medium sweet potatoes
½ cup flour
Salt
½ cup sage leaves

4. Keep the fried sweet potatoes warm on a baking sheet in the oven while frying the remaining batches. (Alternatively, you can roast the potatoes on a baking sheet in the oven at 450°F, though they won't be quite as crispy. If preparing in the oven, be sure not to crowd the potatoes on the baking sheet; none of the potatoes should be touching.)

5. When the sweet potatoes are cooked, add sage to the oil and fry until crisp, about 1 minute. Drain the sage on paper towels and sprinkle over the sweet potato fries.

GINGERY GREEN BEANS

Serves 4 to 6

2 pounds string beans
4 tablespoons olive oil, divided
3 tablespoons minced fresh ginger, divided
6 minced garlic cloves, divided
Sea salt
Lemon wedges, for serving

1. Bring a large pot of salted water to a boil. Fill a large bowl with ice water. Add string beans to the pot and cook over high heat until they're crisp-tender and still have a bright-green color, about 4 minutes.

2. Using tongs or a slotted spoon, transfer the beans to the ice water, then drain them in a colander.

3. Working in two batches, heat half the beans over high heat in a large skillet in 2 tablespoons olive oil, with 1½ tablespoons ginger and 3 minced garlic cloves per batch. Cook for 3 to 4 minutes, until the garlic and ginger soften. Repeat with the second batch. Serve the green beans sprinkled with a dash of sea salt and lemon wedges on the side.

BAKED NEW POTATOES WITH TOPPINGS

1. Preheat the oven to 425°F. In a large saucepan, cover potatoes with 2 inches of cold water and bring to a boil. Cook over high heat until almost tender when pierced with a fork, about 20 minutes.

2. Drain potatoes and cut in half. Spread the potato halves on a large roasting pan and drizzle with olive oil. Sprinkle with salt, a few grinds of pepper, and rosemary, and toss well to coat.

3. Roast for 25 minutes, until golden and completely tender. (Or wrap in aluminum foil and cook on the grill for the same amount of time.)

4. When they're ready, dollop spoonfuls of your favorite topping on the potatoes, or try one of the ideas below:

Serves 4

1 pound medium red bliss potatoes
½ tablespoon olive oil
2 tablespoons sea salt
Freshly ground pepper
Leaves from 2 fresh rosemary sprigs

TOPPING 1

Mix together olives, capers, tuna, lemon juice, olive oil, and salt and pepper to taste.

¼ cup chopped black olives
2 tablespoons capers
1 can olive oil–packed tuna
⅓ cup freshly squeezed lemon juice
½ tablespoon olive oil
Salt and freshly ground pepper

TOPPING 2

1 cup plain yogurt
2 tablespoons minced fresh
  flat-leaf parsley
½ tablespoon crushed garlic
Salt and freshly ground
  pepper

Mix yogurt, parsley, garlic (use a garlic press if you have one), and salt and pepper to taste.

TOPPING 3

2 plum tomatoes, diced
¼ cup minced fresh basil
2 tablespoons olive oil
½ tablespoon minced garlic
Salt and freshly ground
  pepper

Mix tomatoes, basil, olive oil, garlic, and salt and pepper to taste.

TOPPING 4

1 cup grated Cheddar
  cheese
1 tablespoon minced
  scallions
½ tablespoon minced or
  crushed garlic
1 tablespoon minced fresh
  flat-leaf parsley
1 tablespoon unsalted
  butter (softened)
Salt and freshly ground
  pepper

Mix cheese, scallions, garlic, parsley, butter, and salt and pepper to taste.

cheap

&

easy

meals

Clean Out Your Refrigerator Fried Rice

Fried Rice with Bacon and Vegetables

Professional chefs know it, and now you do too: Nothing saves those sad, wilted veggies at the bottom of your crisper like fried rice. (One of our editors always orders an extra carton of rice with her Chinese food so she can do this with it a day or two later.) And while we can't send you fortune cookies with this recipe, we're pretty sure that:

"Good news will be brought to you by mail."
"You are next in line for a promotion in your firm."
"Your first love has never forgotten you."

1. Preheat the oven to 425°F. Line a large rimmed baking sheet with foil. Place the bacon on the prepared sheet and roast on the middle or lower rack for about 12 minutes, until browned and crisp. Let cool, then crumble into bite-size bits.

2. Meanwhile, in a large skillet (the largest one you have), heat the butter over moderate heat until it begins to foam, about 1 minute. Pour in the eggs; turn the heat down to low and cook, stirring often, until just scrambled, about 3 minutes. Transfer to a plate and break up into small pieces.

[CONTINUED]

Serves 4

6 to 8 slices bacon (about half of a 12-ounce package)
1 tablespoon butter
2 large eggs, lightly beaten
2 tablespoons olive oil
3 garlic cloves, minced
½ jalapeño pepper, minced and seeded (it's hotter with seeds)
1 medium onion, diced
1 tablespoon minced fresh ginger
At least 3 of any of the following veggies that you have in the refrigerator or freezer (any combo will do, and the more the better):
2 carrots, grated
1 green bell pepper, sliced
1 red bell pepper, sliced
¾ cup sliced mushrooms
¾ cup diced asparagus
¾ cup frozen peas
¾ cup bean sprouts
¾ cup snap peas
¾ cup snow peas
¾ cup broccoli florets, chopped

1 cup chopped Swiss chard leaves and
stalks

3 cups cooked white or brown rice

¼ cup soy sauce (or more, to taste)

Sriracha or any other hot sauce, to
taste (optional)

3. In the same skillet, heat the oil over moderately high heat. Add the garlic, jalapeño, onion, ginger, and any combination of veggies and cook, stirring often, until softened, about 10 minutes.

4. Add the bacon, eggs, rice, and soy sauce, and cook, stirring constantly, until the rice absorbs the soy sauce and the mixture is heated through. Add more soy sauce to taste. Mix in ¼ to ½ teaspoon Sriracha, if using, or more if you like it spicy. Spoon the rice onto plates and serve.

Hot Date Cool Noodles

Spicy Soba Noodles with Peanut Butter, Cilantro, and Scallions

The trick to a sexy dinner is not slaving over a sweaty stove—it's getting in and out of the kitchen fast. These noodles can be plated in about fifteen minutes flat. And in warm weather, you can stick them in the fridge for twenty minutes before you eat because they also taste great cold.

1. Bring a large pot of water to a boil and add a large pinch of salt. Add the noodles and cook according to package instructions until al dente. Drain.

2. Meanwhile, in a blender or mini food processor, mix the peanut butter, red pepper flakes, honey, lime juice, soy sauce, sesame oil, and 1 tablespoon water.

3. While the noodles are still warm, toss them with the sauce, cilantro, and scallions. Sprinkle with black sesame seeds, if using. Add salt and pepper to taste. Serve warm or chilled.

Serves 2

Salt
One 12-ounce package soba, udon, or
　lo-mein noodles
2 tablespoons peanut butter (either
　chunky or smooth, up to you!)
½ teaspoon red pepper flakes
2 teaspoons honey
2 teaspoons fresh lime juice
1 tablespoon soy sauce
1 tablespoon sesame oil
¼ cup chopped fresh cilantro, or more
　to taste
2 to 3 scallions, chopped
1 teaspoon black sesame seeds
　(optional)
Freshly ground pepper

It's Almost Payday Chili

Meaty Chili Spiked with Jalapeños and Cheese

Serves 6 to 8

1½ teaspoons cumin seeds (or 1 teaspoon ground cumin)

½ cup sour cream

2 tablespoons chopped fresh cilantro

1 tablespoon olive oil

One 1-pound beef chuck roast—fat trimmed, meat cut into 1-inch cubes

2 garlic cloves, minced

1 large yellow onion, diced

1 jalapeño pepper, seeded and minced

1 teaspoon salt

2 tablespoons chili powder

1½ teaspoons dried oregano

One 14-ounce can diced tomatoes, including juice

½ ounce dark chocolate, cut into small pieces

2 ounces goat cheese, crumbled

1½ teaspoons sugar

½ teaspoon ground cinnamon

1½ tablespoons hot sauce, such as Tabasco

Our friend Patrick Fusco perfected this low-cost recipe for a cook-off. It starts with an affordable chuck roast; toasted cumin seeds, chili powder, and jalapeño add layers of expensive-tasting heat; and a smidge of chocolate is a subtle surprise. Even better? This ambitious recipe makes a huge batch—more than enough to share with friends. If you're solo, you can always freeze leftovers once they've cooled.

1. Preheat the oven to 350°F.

2. In a small skillet, toast the cumin seeds over moderate heat until fragrant, about 3 minutes. Transfer to a mortar and pestle or spice grinder, and let cool completely. Finely grind. Skip this step if you're using ground cumin.

3. In a small bowl, mix the sour cream and cilantro. Cover and refrigerate.

4. In a large casserole or Dutch oven fitted with a lid, add the olive oil and beef and cook over moderate heat, turning occasionally, until well browned, about 8 minutes. Add the garlic, onion, and jalapeño, and cook, stirring often, until the onion is just translucent, about 6 minutes. Add the ground cumin, salt, chili powder, oregano, and tomatoes with juice, and bring to a simmer.

5. Cover the casserole and transfer to the oven. Bake, about 2 hours, stirring occasionally, until the meat is tender when pierced with a fork.

6. Stir in the chocolate, cheese, sugar, cinnamon, and hot sauce. Simmer on the stove for 10 minutes to let the spices incorporate. Serve the chili in bowls, with a dollop of cilantro sour cream on top.

glamour girl tip

Be careful when cutting jalapeños! Wear latex gloves to protect your hands, or else make sure not to bring your jalapeño-spiced fingers anywhere near your eyes. Even after washing your hands, you still risk stinging your eyes with the jalapeño residue several hours after you touch the peppers.

Pauper's Fish Feast

Lime Tilapia

Serves 4

4 tablespoons (½ stick) unsalted
 butter, softened
1 scallion, finely chopped
2 tablespoons finely chopped fresh
 cilantro
1 teaspoon finely grated lime zest
2 teaspoons fresh lime juice
1 teaspoon salt
Four 5- to 6-ounce skinless tilapia
 fillets (or lemon sole or flounder)
2 tablespoons vegetable oil
Cooked basmati rice, lime wedges,
 and chopped peanuts, for serving
 (optional)

If you're looking for a handy way to make your paycheck disappear, enter a seafood restaurant. They're money pits, which is a shame, considering the fact that *some* types of fish—like tilapia—really needn't be expensive at all. This recipe is a satisfying substitute for a meal out. It makes great fish tacos too (perfect for a party at your place). Invite your friends over, bank what you would have spent dining out, and watch your balance grow.

1. In a small bowl, mix the butter, scallion, cilantro, lime zest, lime juice, and ½ teaspoon salt.

2. Pat the fish dry and sprinkle with the remaining ½ teaspoon salt. In a large nonstick skillet, heat 1 tablespoon oil over moderately high heat. Add 2 fish fillets and cook, turning once, until golden and just cooked through, 4 to 5 minutes. Transfer to a plate.

3. Put a dollop of the lime-cilantro butter on each piece of fish while it's still hot, and cover the plate to keep warm. Cook the remaining fish. Serve over rice with lime wedges on the side and peanuts sprinkled on top, if desired. For fish tacos, slice the fillets and place on small flour tortillas. Sprinkle with sliced red onions, and serve with sour cream, lime wedges, and salsa.

Single-Digit Grocery Bill Stew

Beef Stew with Potatoes in Tomato and Thyme Broth

If you've been building your pantry with our essential groceries (see page 256), then all you'll need to make this hearty dish is an inexpensive cut of beef and some of the humblest items in the produce aisle. The longer you let this stew, the better it gets.

1 pound beef chuck roast, cut into
  2-inch pieces
Salt and freshly ground pepper
1 tablespoon olive oil
5 carrots—1 quartered, 4 thinly sliced
  into matchsticks
1 celery stalk, quartered
1 medium onion, quartered
3 garlic cloves
One 8-ounce can tomato sauce
2 tablespoons balsamic vinegar
One 14-ounce can low-sodium beef
  broth
1 bay leaf
2 thyme sprigs
1 pound small white or red boiling
  potatoes, quartered (with the peel
  on or off)
Cooked rice, buttered noodles, or
  crusty bread, for serving (optional)

1. Pat the meat dry and season with 1 teaspoon salt and ¼ teaspoon pepper. In a large pot, heat the oil over moderately high heat until it shimmers. Working in two batches, add the meat and cook, turning occasionally, until richly browned all over, about 8 minutes. Transfer the meat to a bowl.

2. Turn the heat down to moderate, then add the quartered carrot, celery, onion, and garlic to the pot. Cook, stirring occasionally, until well browned, about 10 minutes. Stir in the tomato sauce and cook for 2 minutes, then stir in the vinegar and cook for 2 minutes.

3. Add the broth, beef, bay leaf, and thyme. Turn the heat up to high and bring to a boil. Cover, turn the heat down to low, and simmer until the meat is very tender, about 2 hours.

4. Set a colander in a large bowl. Pour the stew into the colander. Return the meat to the pot along with the liquid in the bowl. Discard the remaining solids in the colander.

[CONTINUED]

5. Add the potatoes and sliced carrots to the pot with the beef and liquid, stirring to submerge them. Simmer, uncovered, stirring occasionally, until the potatoes and carrots are tender, about 25 minutes. Serve with rice, buttered noodles, or crusty bread, if desired.

glamour girl tip

This stew improves in flavor if made at least 1 day ahead. Once it cools, cover and refrigerate for up to 5 days.

Frugalista Burritos

Bean-Stuffed Tortillas with Cheese and Avocado

Our staff still mourns the disappearance of NYC's many Burritoville restaurants, which churned out tasty $7 burritos. So we invented our own at-home interpretation (which, incidentally, costs *less* than the original). This simple, spicy, one-handed meal is take-out quick, too.

1. Preheat the oven to 350°F. Wrap the flour tortillas together in foil and heat in the oven 8 to 10 minutes while making the burrito filling. They should still be soft and easy to bend when you remove them from the oven. Keep the oven on for step 3, if desired.

2. In a large skillet, heat the oil over moderate heat. Add the onion and cook, stirring often, until golden and softened, about 10 minutes. Add the chipotles with sauce, tomato, and beans and cook, stirring, until heated through, about 5 minutes. Add salt and pepper to taste.

3. Lay the warm tortillas on a work surface and spread the lower thirds of each with ¼ cup rice (if using), ½ cup or more of the bean mixture, ¼ cup cheese, some avocado slices, and chopped cilantro. Gently mix the ingredients together with a knife to blend. Roll up the tortillas to form burritos, folding

Serves 2

2 large (10- to 12-inch) flour tortillas
2 tablespoons vegetable oil
½ cup chopped onion
1 tablespoon chopped chipotles in adobo from a can, including sauce
½ cup chopped tomato
One 16-ounce can pinto beans, rinsed
Salt and freshly ground pepper
½ cup cooked white or brown rice (optional), heated in the microwave
½ cup grated Monterey Jack cheese
1 ripe avocado, quartered, pitted, peeled, and sliced
¼ cup chopped fresh cilantro
Sour cream, hot sauce, and/or salsa for serving (optional)

in the sides as you go. Put the burritos back in the hot oven for 3 to 4 minutes, so the cheese melts, if desired. Serve the burritos immediately, with sour cream, hot sauce, and/or salsa on the side.

glamour girl tip

Don't be afraid to get your hands a little dirty when rolling up your burrito (why do you think those guys wear plastic gloves?). The more you manhandle it, the less likely your fillings will fall out.

Lazy Day Frittata

Fluffy Ham and Cheese Frittata

You know those cooks who make omelet flipping look so easy? Show-offs. The next time you're craving a simple meal of eggs but don't have the energy to attempt any one-handed, gravity-defying tricks, this frittata is as versatile as an omelet—perfect with whatever combination of meat, cheese, veggies, or herbs you have handy, but lighter and fluffier when it cooks up. The pielike slices are pretty on your plate, especially with a green salad on the side for a light dinner. Consider it a thrifty woman's dream.

Serves 4

2 tablespoons olive oil
½ cup chopped onion
1 cup chopped pancetta, smoked ham, or cooked sausage
½ cup chopped red or green bell pepper (optional)
8 large eggs
¼ cup half-and-half
Salt and freshly ground black pepper
¼ cup crumbled goat or feta cheese (or freshly grated mozzarella, Cheddar, or Gruyère cheese)

1. Preheat the broiler and position the oven rack 6 inches from the heat. In a 12-inch cast-iron skillet, heat the olive oil over moderate heat. Cook the onion, stirring a few times, until translucent and soft, about 4 minutes.

2. Add the pancetta and red or green bell pepper (if using). Cook, stirring a few times, until the pancetta is slightly browned around the edges and the pepper is just tender, about 4 minutes.

3. In a medium bowl, whisk together the eggs, half-and-half, and a pinch each of salt and pepper. Pour the egg mixture into the skillet. Stir to incorporate the fillings evenly

and cook until the bottom is set, about 9 minutes. Sprinkle the cheese on top.

4. Place the skillet under the broiler. Broil for about 3 minutes, until the top is set. Cut into slices and serve.

glamour girl tip

Once you have the method down, try experimenting with different filling combinations instead of—or in addition to—the ham and cheese. We like chopped jalapeños, tomatoes, and Cheddar; diced potatoes and bacon; salami and ricotta; broccoli rabe and Parmesan.

Broke and Fabulous Grilled Cheese

Crusty Grilled Cheese Sandwiches, with Variations

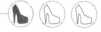

When you're watching your budget but not willing to succumb to cereal for dinner (again), this simple sandwich is the way to go. It's an update on the kids' menu classic; it calls for sourdough and Cheddar instead of white bread and Kraft singles—but it still requires nothing more than bread, butter, and cheese. The key is buttering the *outside* of the bread—all the way to the edge—so that you get that golden-brown crispy finish. And grating the cheese rather than slicing means it will do that stringy, melty thing when you bite into it. If you've got an apple lying around, try the honey and apple version below. It's a sweet/savory home run.

Serves 2

1 tablespoon butter, softened
4 slices sourdough, rye, or other bread
1 cup grated Cheddar cheese

1. Spread the butter on one side of each slice of bread, making sure the butter reaches all the way to the edges. Set 2 slices on a work surface, buttered sides down, and mound the unbuttered sides with ½ cup grated cheese each. Set the remaining bread slices on the cheese, buttered sides up, and press together.

2. Heat a large cast-iron skillet over moderate heat. Put the sandwiches in the skillet and cook until the undersides are browned, about 3 minutes. Turn the sandwiches over and cook until the second side is browned and the cheese is melted, about 3 minutes longer. Cut the sandwiches in two and serve.

[CONTINUED]

VARIATIONS:

- Top the cheese with crisp bacon and slices of tomato and avocado.
- Spread the insides of the bread with honey and top the cheese with thin slices of green apple.
- Use crumbled blue cheese instead of Cheddar, and top with a sprinkling of chopped smoked almonds and thin slices of pear.
- Spread the insides of the bread with grainy mustard, use Gruyère cheese, and top with thin slices of Black Forest or honey-baked ham.

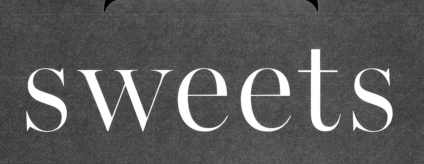

sweets

BFF Birthday Cake

Vanilla Layer Cake with Chocolate Buttercream Frosting

A great friend deserves an even greater cake, and this one delivers on all levels. It's not much more time consuming than the box kind, but the end result is definitely worth the effort. The cake bakes up moist and buttery, and the icing is inspired—you make it using marshmallow fluff instead of sugar, which gives a light, mousselike consistency. (Pop Rocks on top bring the fun.) Oh, and it's chocolate. Let the candle licking begin!

1. Make the cake: Preheat the oven to 350°F. Butter and flour two 9-inch cake pans.

2. In a large bowl, sift together the flour, baking powder, baking soda, and salt.

3. Using a stand mixer or a hand mixer, in another large bowl beat the 2 sticks butter and the sugar until light and fluffy. Beat in the vanilla. Add the eggs, one at a time, beating well between additions. Beat in the buttermilk.

4. Add the flour mixture in 4 batches, beating between additions until it is just combined, being careful not to overmix.

[CONTINUED]

Serves 12 to 15

VANILLA LAYER CAKE
2 sticks unsalted butter, plus more
  for buttering the cake pans
4 cups all-purpose flour, plus more for
  dusting the cake pans
2 teaspoons baking powder
1 teaspoon baking soda
1½ teaspoons salt
2 cups sugar
2 tablespoons pure vanilla extract
4 large eggs, at room temperature
2 cups buttermilk, at room
  temperature

CHOCOLATE BUTTERCREAM-
MARSHMALLOW FROSTING
2 sticks unsalted butter, at room
  temperature
Two 7.5-ounce jars marshmallow
  cream
¾ cup cocoa powder
⅔ cup semisweet chocolate chips,
  melted and cooled (for directions on
  how to melt chocolate, see page 233)

1 tablespoon pure vanilla extract

1 package strawberry-flavored Pop
Rocks (optional)

5. Divide the batter between 2 cake pans. Bake for about 35 minutes, or until a toothpick inserted in the center comes out clean. Run a knife gently between each cake and the edge of the pan. Lightly shake the pan up and down to loosen the cake, then slowly tip the pan over until the cake starts to come out. Support the cake with your other hand and forearm as you take it out of the pan, then tip the cake back so it stays right side up. Put the cake on an elevated wire rack (so it can air on all sides and not get too moist on the bottom).

6. Meanwhile, make the frosting: Using a stand mixer or hand mixer, in a large bowl, beat the butter until fluffy. Beat in the marshmallow cream until smooth. Add the cocoa powder, melted chocolate, and vanilla and beat until incorporated. The frosting should be smooth and spreadable; if the mixture is too thick, mix in 1 tablespoon water.

7. When the cake layers are completely cool, place one layer on a cake stand or plate. Spread frosting on top. Place the second cake layer on the frosting and finish frosting the cake sides and top. Immediately before serving, sprinkle the top with a few Pop Rocks here and there, if desired.

glamour girl tip

Using an offset spatula (a spatula with a blade that bends upward) helps transfer cakes neatly from the pan to a cake stand. You can also run the spatula under hot water and use it to smooth out the frosting.

Impress His Family Chardonnay Cake

Creamy White Bundt Cake with Chardonnay Glaze

This cake is sophisticated (the wine does that) but bake-sale simple. It tells his parents, "I know how to take care of the people I love." And you do!

Serves 10

1. Make the cake: Preheat the oven to 350°F. Grease and flour a Bundt pan or a 9-by-9-inch pan, shaking off any excess flour. Set aside.

2. With a stand mixer or hand mixer, in a large bowl, beat together the butter, sugar, eggs, pudding mix, chardonnay, milk, and vanilla until well combined. In a medium bowl, whisk together the flour, salt, and baking powder. Add the dry ingredients to the wet ingredients and mix just until combined. If it looks a little lumpy due to specks of butter, that's okay; do not overmix.

3. Scrape the batter into the prepared pan. Bake for about 50 minutes, or until the edges of the cake appear light golden and a toothpick inserted into the center comes out clean.

4. Meanwhile, make the glaze: In a medium saucepan, combine all the ingredients and bring to a boil. Reduce the heat to low and let simmer for about 10 minutes, until the mixture reduces by one fourth.

[CONTINUED]

CAKE

2 sticks unsalted butter, melted and cooled to room temperature, plus more for buttering the pan

2 cups sugar

4 large eggs, at room temperature

One 3.5-ounce package regular or instant vanilla pudding mix

½ cup chardonnay or another medium or full-bodied white wine, such as Chablis or Viognier

1 cup whole milk, warmed in the microwave for about 20 seconds

1 teaspoon pure vanilla extract

3 cups cake flour or all-purpose flour, plus more for dusting the pan

½ teaspoon salt

2 teaspoons baking powder

GLAZE

4 tablespoons unsalted butter (½ stick)

1 cup sugar

¼ cup chardonnay or other dry white wine

5. When the cake has finished baking, remove it from the oven and pierce it several times with a skewer or carving fork. Immediately pour the hot glaze onto the pan and let stand for about 15 minutes, until the glaze has been absorbed.

6. If using a Bundt pan, carefully turn it over onto a plate and tap the edges a bit. The cake should glide out easily. Serve immediately. Save a slice or two to enjoy with coffee the next morning.

Mea Culpa Cheesecake

Creamy Cheesecake with Cookie-Crumb Crust

You don't have to be a Real Housewife of Anywhere to find your-self involved in some serious friend drama every now and then. So do the classy thing you never see on reality TV: Make amends. Bake up this wow factor cheesecake, serve it to anyone you've wronged, and all will be right with your world.

1. Preheat the oven to 325°F.

2. Make the crust: In a bowl, mix the crumbs and butter with a fork until well blended. Scrape the crumb mixture into an 8-inch square or a 9-inch round springform pan (see Note). Using the back of a spoon or your fingers, press the crumbs into a ¼-inch layer onto the bottom and up the sides of the pan to within 1 inch of the top. Refrigerate for 20 minutes, or until set.

3. Make the filling: In a large mixing bowl, with the mixer at medium speed, beat the cream cheese until smooth. Add the remaining ingredients and beat until just blended. Scrape the cream cheese filling into the crumb-lined pan. Bake for about 1 hour and 20 minutes, or until lightly golden on top.

Serves 12

CRUST

1 cup crushed graham crackers or
   crisp chocolate cookies
6 tablespoons butter, melted

FILLING

Four 8-ounce packages cream cheese,
   at room temperature
6 large eggs, at room temperature
1¾ cups sugar
⅛ teaspoon salt
1 teaspoon pure vanilla extract

TOPPING (OPTIONAL)

2 cups raspberries, sliced strawberries,
   or sliced kiwi, or berries with port
   (see recipe, page 237)

[CONTINUED]

4. Turn off the oven and let the cake stand in the oven for 1 hour.

5. Remove the cake from the oven and set the pan on a wire rack. Run a sharp, thin knife between the cheesecake and the side of the pan to prevent it from cracking once it has chilled. Let cool completely. Cover the cake with aluminum foil and chill overnight before serving.

6. To serve, garnish the cake with raspberries, overlapping slices of strawberry or kiwi, or berries with port.

NOTE: A springform pan has removable sides, so you can keep the cake anchored to the bottom of the pan while you pop the sides out. It's particularly helpful for cheesecake—a dessert so delicate it can otherwise break as you're removing it from the pan.

You Rock Cupcakes

Frosted Vanilla Cupcakes

The great British writer Iris Murdoch believed that "One of the secrets to a happy life is continuous small treats." These cupcakes are the perfect small treats; you may just find yourself making them continuously.

Makes 18 cupcakes

2 cups all-purpose flour

2 teaspoons baking powder

¾ teaspoon salt

1 cup whole milk

1 teaspoon pure vanilla extract

1¼ sticks unsalted butter, softened (10 tablespoons)

1¼ cups sugar

3 large eggs

1. Preheat the oven to 350°F. Line 18 muffin cups with paper liners.

2. In a large bowl, whisk together the flour, baking powder, and salt. In a medium bowl, stir together the milk and vanilla. Set both aside.

3. In another large bowl with an electric mixer at medium speed, beat the butter and sugar until fluffy, about 5 minutes. Add in the eggs, one at a time, beating well after each addition, until smooth and evenly incorporated.

4. With the mixer on low, add the flour mixture in two batches, alternating with the milk mixture, until just combined. Divide the batter evenly into the cups. Bake for 20 to 24 minutes, until a toothpick inserted into the center of a cupcake comes out clean. Cool completely before removing from the muffin cups or frosting (see next page for frosting variations).

[CONTINUED]

BASIC VANILLA BUTTER FROSTING

Makes 2⅓ cups

2 sticks unsalted butter, softened

One 16-ounce package confectioners' sugar

4 tablespoons milk, at room temperature

1 teaspoon pure vanilla extract

¼ teaspoon salt

In a large bowl with an electric mixer at medium speed, beat the butter, sugar, and 2 tablespoons milk for 3 to 5 minutes until smooth and free of lumps and graininess. Add the vanilla and salt, then beat in additional milk as needed for a creamy frosting.

VARIATION: CHOCOLATE BUTTER FROSTING

Prepare the above recipe, but add ⅓ cup unsweetened cocoa with the butter and sugar, and beat in 4 ounces bittersweet chocolate, melted and cooled.

Hers and His Cupcakes

Chocolate and Dark Beer Cupcakes with Irish Cream Frosting

Glance at the ingredient list and you'll see why these little darlings are a unisex hit. Beer! Baileys! Butter! Cocoa! There's something for everyone, and when you mix it all together, the result is rich and chocolaty, with just a hint of booze.

Makes 10 cupcakes

CUPCAKES

½ cup Guinness or other dark beer, porter, or stout
4 tablespoons unsalted butter
6 tablespoons unsweetened cocoa
1 cup all-purpose flour
1 cup sugar
¾ teaspoon baking soda
¼ teaspoon salt
1 large egg
⅓ cup sour cream
Irish Cream Frosting (recipe follows)

1. Preheat the oven to 350°F. Line 10 muffin cups with 10 muffin liners.

2. In a medium saucepan, combine the beer and butter. Bring to a boil, then immediately reduce to a simmer. Add the cocoa and whisk until smooth. Remove from the heat and set aside.

3. In a medium bowl, whisk together the flour, sugar, baking soda, and salt. Set aside.

4. In a large bowl, whisk together the egg and sour cream until smooth. Whisk in the beer mixture.

5. Fold the flour mixture into the batter until just combined.

6. Spoon the batter into the muffin cups, filling them three-quarters full. Bake for about 20 minutes, or until a toothpick comes out clean.

[CONTINUED]

7. When the cupcakes are cool, spread the frosting over them. Serve.

IRISH CREAM FROSTING

4 tablespoons unsalted butter, at
    room temperature

1½ cups confectioners' sugar

1½ tablespoons Irish cream, such as
    Baileys (more optional)

1 to 2 tablespoons milk (optional)

Using a stand mixer or hand mixer, beat the butter until light and fluffy. With the motor on low, add the sugar, ½ cup at a time, beating between additions until smooth. Beat in the Irish cream. The mixture should be smooth and spreadable; if it is too thick, add 1 to 2 tablespoons milk or Baileys to thin it out.

glamour girl tip

Open your calendar to March 17 and write "make chocolate and beer cupcakes." While this dessert is good any day of the week, it's too Irish not to enjoy on St. Patty's Day as well. *Sláinte!*

Hook Him Apple Pie

Classic Apple Pie with Buttery Crust

When *Glamour* reader Laura Wheeler made Engagement Chicken for her guy, she topped it off with a recipe she'd invented herself: Hook Him Apple Pie. The one-two punch worked: He proposed. We love Laura's spicy, saucy, apple-packed filling (she prebakes it to thicken and draw out the flavors), and have added our own buttery, sugary crust. The pie's charms work on aunts, landladies, and cubicle mates too—anyone you're sweet on.

1. **Make the filling: Preheat the oven to 400°F. Butter a 3-quart baking dish.**

2. **In a large bowl, combine the apples with the sugars, cornstarch, salt, and spices and stir to coat thoroughly. Stir in the melted butter and lemon juice.**

3. **Cover the baking dish with foil and cut large vents in the foil. Bake for 35 minutes. Remove the foil, stir the apples, and let cool to room temperature.**

4. **Make the pie crust: Combine the flour and salt in a food processor. Quickly cut the cold butter into small pieces, being careful not to warm it with your hands, and add it to the flour mixture.**

[CONTINUED]

Serves 6

FILLING

8 to 10 apples (Golden Delicious, Pink Lady, Granny Smith, and Fuji are good choices), peeled, cored, and sliced ¼-inch thick (8 cups)

½ cup firmly packed light brown sugar

½ cup granulated sugar

3 tablespoons cornstarch

½ teaspoon salt

1 teaspoon ground cinnamon

½ teaspoon apple pie spice (or ¼ teaspoon ground nutmeg, ⅛ teaspoon ground allspice, and ⅛ teaspoon ground cardamom)

4 tablespoons unsalted butter, melted

2 tablespoons fresh lemon juice

PIE CRUST

2½ cups all-purpose flour

½ teaspoon salt

2 sticks unsalted butter, cold

6 to 8 tablespoons cold water (it should be ice cold)

1 egg, beaten with 2 tablespoons water

½ teaspoon sugar, for dusting

5. Pulse the flour mixture in short blasts (5 seconds each) until the butter bits are about the size of peanuts or hazelnuts. Add 6 tablespoons ice water and continue to pulse in short blasts until incorporated. Check the consistency of the mixture by squeezing it in your hands. If it is floury and doesn't hold together, drizzle in a bit more ice water and pulse again. As soon as the dough holds together, remove it from the processor and place on a lightly floured surface. Divide the dough in half and roll each half into a ball, then press into a disc, cover with plastic wrap, and place in the refrigerator to rest for an hour.

6. Remove the first ball of dough from the refrigerator (leave the second one in the refrigerator until you are ready for it) and roll out on a lightly floured surface until it's 12 inches in diameter (it helps to rotate the dough between rolls, and to flip it occasionally, dusting as necessary with a little more flour to avoid sticking). Place the dough in a 9-inch pie pan, pressing gently along the base and sides of the pan. Add the cooled apple mixture. Then repeat the dough-rolling steps with the second ball of dough and place it over the apple filling. Trim the dough so only about ½ inch is hanging over, then turn the edges under and crimp them with your fingers.

7. Cut vents in the top crust. Brush some of the egg mixture over the center of the pie. Cover the edges with aluminum foil and dust the pie lightly with sugar.

8. Bake 20 minutes. Remove the foil and bake until the crust is golden, 20 to 30 minutes more. Let cool to warm or room temperature before slicing.

Make New Friends Plum Cobbler

Fresh-Baked Cobbler with Ripe Plums and Sweet Buttermilk Crust

Glamour executive editor Lauren Brody got this recipe from her Grandma Dolores. When Lauren and her husband go out to dinner with new friends, they like to invite them back to their place for dessert. (The cobbler can be made ahead of time and reheated.) This sweet, tart goodness says, "Let's be friends," without trying too hard. The last time Lauren made it, she sent the leftovers home with her guests (bonus points!) and had this e-mail in her inbox the next morning: "Just finished the cobbler for breakfast—amazing!"

Serves 8

8 to 10 firm-ripe plums, halved, pitted and cut into ⅛-inch slices (3 cups)

¾ cup sugar, plus 1 teaspoon for dusting

1 teaspoon ground cinnamon

1 teaspoon pure vanilla extract

1 cup all-purpose flour

2 teaspoons baking powder

¼ teaspoon baking soda

¼ teaspoon salt

Scant ½ cup buttermilk or whole milk

4 tablespoons (½ stick) unsalted butter, melted and cooled to room temperature

Vanilla ice cream, for serving (optional)

1. Preheat the oven to 400°F. In a medium bowl, mix the plums, ¼ cup sugar, cinnamon, and vanilla until combined. Spoon into a 1½- to 2-quart ceramic or glass baking dish. Set aside.

2. In another bowl, whisk the flour, baking powder, baking soda, salt, and ½ cup sugar. Add the buttermilk and melted butter and mix just until combined, being careful not to overmix.

[CONTINUED]

3. Using a large spoon, dollop the batter on the plums until all the batter is used up. (Don't worry about covering the entire surface—the batter will spread when it bakes.)

4. Bake for 25 to 35 minutes, or until the cobbler topping is golden and set. Remove from the oven and immediately sprinkle the top with 1 teaspoon sugar. Serve warm, topped with a scoop of vanilla ice cream, if desired.

Bribe a Kid Brownies

Rich, Chocolate Brownies

Your nephew. Your boss's daughter. Your boyfriend's kid from his first marriage. When new children enter your life, make these brownies to sweet-tooth your way into their world.

Makes nine 2½-inch-square brownies

Three 1-ounce squares unsweetened baking chocolate
1 stick unsalted butter
2 large eggs
1 cup sugar
¾ teaspoon pure vanilla extract
½ cup all-purpose flour

1. Preheat the oven to 400°F. Grease an 8-by-8-inch glass or ceramic baking pan.

2. In a double boiler set over simmering water, melt the chocolate and butter. (If you don't have a double boiler, place the chocolate and butter in a metal mixing bowl over a pot of barely simmering water, making sure not to get water into the chocolate mix.) Remove the melted chocolate mixture from the heat and let cool slightly.

3. In a large bowl with a mixer at medium speed, beat the eggs until smooth. Gradually add the sugar, beating until very thick and pale yellow, about 6 minutes. Add the vanilla and melted chocolate mixture and stir until blended.

4. Gently fold in the flour until just combined. Scrape the batter into the prepared pan. Bake for 14 to 16 minutes, until a toothpick inserted in the center has moist crumbs attached. Don't overbake; brownies should be very moist. Remove the pan from the oven, place it on a wire rack, and let cool completely. Cut into nine 2¹/₂-inch squares and serve.

Win Friends and Influence People Cookies

Chocolate-Chocolate Chip Cookies

Makes about 48 cookies

1¼ cups all-purpose flour

¾ cup unsweetened cocoa

¾ teaspoon baking soda

1¼ teaspoons salt

2 sticks unsalted butter (1 cup), softened

1 cup packed light brown sugar

½ cup granulated sugar

2 large eggs

1½ teaspoons pure vanilla extract

One 12-ounce package semisweet or
 bittersweet chocolate chips (2 cups)

1 cup coarsely chopped walnuts
 (optional)

There are a few things that every woman who loves to cook should have up her sleeve: a go-to dinner for guests, an easy solo meal, a signature cocktail, and a take-anywhere dessert. If you haven't yet mastered a sweet treat, may we suggest this chocolaty chocolate chip cookie recipe? Bring a batch of these anywhere and watch the goodwill follow.

1. Preheat the oven to 375°F. Position the racks in the upper and lower thirds of the oven.

2. In a medium bowl, whisk together the flour, cocoa, baking soda, and salt.

3. In a large bowl, with a mixer on high speed, beat the butter and sugars until light and fluffy, about 4 minutes.

4. Beat in the eggs, one at a time. Mix in the vanilla until combined. Add the flour mixture and combine thoroughly. Stir in the chocolate chips and walnuts (if using).

5. Drop rounded tablespoons of the mixture onto ungreased baking sheets about 2 inches apart. Bake for about 8 minutes, until puffy and the bottoms are golden brown. Let cool on baking sheets about 2 minutes, then transfer them to wire racks to cool completely.

Fancy Pants Coffee and Ice Cream Sundae

Traditional Italian Affogato

Once you've discovered the Italian treat affogato—a grown-up sundae in which vanilla ice cream is covered with espresso and, if you're interested, liqueur—it'll become your go-to dessert for dinner parties. Chilling the espresso requires a little forethought, but once that's done the rest is *molto facile*.

Serves 4

1 pint vanilla or hazelnut ice cream (or gelato)
½ cup brewed espresso, cooled to room temperature or chilled
Liqueur, such as Grand Marnier, crème de cacao, or Kahlùa (optional)
Roughly ground espresso beans, for garnish (optional)

1. Fill four bowls or parfait cups with 2 to 3 scoops each of ice cream, and drizzle each with a quarter of the espresso.

2. Drizzle with liqueur, if using.

3. Garnish with crushed espresso beans, if using.

glamour girl tip

If you don't have an electric espresso maker, you can brew espresso in a stovetop espresso maker or use an electric drip coffee machine: Brew ½ cup ground espresso beans with 3 cups water.

Secretly Good for You Banana Soft Serve

"Ice Cream" with Cocoa Sprinkles

Serves 1 to 2

2 to 3 frozen peeled bananas, broken
into pieces

Cocoa powder or ground cinnamon,
for sprinkling (optional)

Fresh berries, chopped nuts, whipped
cream, or your favorite liqueur
(optional)

We know what you're thinking. How can you make ice cream without ice? Or cream? Or *sugar*? Well, you can't exactly. But you *can* make something that tastes so close no one will know the difference. And when you tell them that the decadent dessert they're swooning over is actually just a frozen banana pureed into oblivion (a classic vegan "ice cream" trick), they will think you're a culinary genius. No need to correct them.

1. In a food processor, process the bananas for about 5 minutes, stopping a few times to scrape down the sides. As each minute passes, the bananas will get light and fluffy, and take on a creamy texture—sort of like soft serve!

2. Scrape the banana "ice cream" into serving bowls. For an extra flavor kick, sprinkle a bit of cocoa powder or cinnamon on top, or get creative by adding other toppings such as berries, chopped nuts, whipped cream, and/or a drizzle of your favorite liqueur.

Get Over Him Berry Parfait

Sweet Mixed Berries with Port

These are better for you than fudge and less dangerous than a drink-and-dial cocktail. When your heart needs mending, consider this recipe your one-bowl support group. It's also great spooned over cold, creamy, comforting scoops of vanilla ice cream.

Serves 2

1 cup mixed berries
3 tablespoons port wine
1 tablespoon sugar (optional)

1. In a small bowl, combine the berries, port wine, and sugar (if using), and toss to coat.

2. Cover and refrigerate for 1 hour, stirring a few times, until the berries have released their juices. Serve in parfait or martini glasses.

glamour girl tip

In addition to ice cream, these berries also work nicely as a topping for Greek yogurt or cheesecake (see recipe, page 223).

'Tis the Season Peppermint Bark

Holiday Chocolate-Peppermint Candy

Makes about 2 pounds bark, enough for around 10 people if you're serving it at a party or about 4 small gift bags if you're making it to give away for the holidays

10 ounces peppermint hard candies or
  6 large candy canes
Cooking spray
12 ounces milk chocolate chips or
  coarsely chopped bar
12 ounces white chocolate chips or
  coarsely chopped bar

Wrap these up in a stiff clear plastic bag (buy at craft stores or online), tie with a red grosgrain ribbon, and you've got a holiday party hostess gift that will knock the stockings off any candle or bouquet or bottle of wine. Especially that regifted merlot your friend Katie just walked in with. Hello, Katie? Didn't we just bring that same bottle to your house last week?

1. Place the candy in a sturdy plastic freezer bag and tap with a hammer or rolling pin until crushed. (This might be noisy!) Alternatively, crush the candy in a food processor.

2. Line a large rimmed sheet with foil and lightly coat with cooking spray. In a double boiler or metal mixing bowl set over barely simmering water, melt the milk chocolate.

3. When the chocolate is nearly melted, remove from the heat and stir until smooth. Pour the chocolate onto the foil-lined pan, and spread with a spatula to form a layer about 1/8 inch thick. Refrigerate until hard, about 30 minutes. Clean the spatula.

4. Meanwhile, repeat step 2 with the white chocolate. When smooth, stir in half the crushed candy. Spoon the white chocolate mixture over the hardened milk chocolate. Spread with

the spatula to form another layer about ⅛ inch thick that covers the milk chocolate layer. Sprinkle the remaining candy on top of the white chocolate.

5. Refrigerate until hard, about 1 hour. When the chocolate has set, peel off the foil, break the bark into pieces, and refrigerate.

NOTE: In step 5, you can freeze the bark for 20 to 30 minutes instead of refrigerating it, to speed up the setting process.

kitchen basics:
How to Serve Fruit for Dessert

After a big meal, sometimes the sweetest, most satisfying treat is a colorful, glorious bowl of juicy, fragrant fruit, ideally grown locally and in season. And one of the greatest things about fruit is that it's fabulous on its own; present a few different fruits in one big bowl on a dinner table, or put different fruits in little bowls and let guests pick their favorites—or try one of our serving suggestions:

FRUIT	WHAT TO LOOK FOR	HOW TO STORE IT	SERVING SUGGESTION
Apricots	Look for fruits that are firm to the touch with a glowing golden-yellow color. Stronger color means sweeter fruit.	Refrigerate and serve as soon as possible. Wash just before using.	Slice apricots into bowls, drizzle with honey, and top with chopped almonds.
Blackberries	Seek out bright, shiny berries without green spots. No stems means a richer, fuller flavor.	Keep, unwashed, in a covered container and use within a day or two. Rinse gently before serving.	Place in bowls with a dollop of whipped cream, and sprinkle grated orange peel on top.
Cherries	Choose firm cherries dark in color (they'll be sweetest). Stems should be green and healthy-looking.	Keep, unwashed, in the refrigerator in sealed plastic bags, and use within three days. Wash just before serving.	Pit and slice the cherries, and fold them into softened vanilla ice cream.
Figs	Pick figs that are soft to the touch, with unblemished, unbruised skin. (A sour odor means they're overripe.)	Use within three days, and rinse gently before serving.	Ripe figs really don't need much else; they can be eaten peeled or whole. You can also halve them and drape them with a thin slice of prosciutto for a sweet-and-savory snack.

FRUIT	WHAT TO LOOK FOR	HOW TO STORE IT	SERVING SUGGESTION
Kiwi	Choose kiwi that feels firm to the touch with no bruises or wrinkles.	Keep at room temperature, stored in a plastic bag, to ripen for a day or so (or till it feels soft to the touch), or store in the refrigerator for up to three days.	Slice kiwi, drizzle with honey, and add a dollop of yogurt and some crushed walnuts on top.
Peaches	Look for skin with a reddish blush on a creamy yellow background. Pick plump, medium-size peaches.	Store at room temperature for three to four days to ripen fully, then keep in sealed plastic bags in the refrigerator for one to two days. Wash gently before serving.	Slice peaches, sprinkle with sugar, and broil in the oven or a toaster oven for a few minutes. Serve with vanilla ice cream.
Plums	Choose plums that are firm with still a little give when you press on them. Look for glossy skin and uniform color (reddish or purple).	If they're ripe, keep in sealed plastic bags in the refrigerator. If they need to ripen, keep them at room temperature for a day, then store in the refrigerator for three to five days. Wash just before serving.	Slice and serve with a piece of your favorite blue cheese (such as Gorgonzola) on the side.
Raspberries	Look for firm, plump berries with uniform color and stems on.	Keep, unwashed, in the refrigerator, and eat the same day or by the next day at the latest. Rinse gently just before serving.	Serve in a bowl with a dollop of whipped cream and a few thin slices of fresh mint on top.
Strawberries	Those big, plump supermarket strawberries tend to be somewhat flavorless. Ignore them in favor of extra-sweet, small, wild strawberries, grown locally and in season, if you can find them.	Keep, unwashed, in the refrigerator and serve the same day or by the next day. Rinse gently just before serving.	Serve in a bowl sprinkled with confectioners' sugar and topped with a dollop of whipped cream. Heaven.

241

menus

for occasions

big & small

Engagement Chicken Dinner

This. Is. It. We have suggested some simple sides that don't overpower The Chicken, but this menu is truly yours to personalize. Start with a cocktail, and switch to wine with the main course. With more than 60 weddings and counting... we've got a good feeling about this.

Classic Manhattans with Maraschino Cherries, PAGE 72

Roasted Cherry Tomatoes, Spinach, and Gorgonzola Cheese Salad, PAGE 96

Engagement Chicken with Lemon and Herbs, PAGE 18

Baked New Potatoes, PAGE 197

Creamy White Bundt Cake with Chardonnay Glaze, PAGE 221

Prove You're Not a Girly-Girl Dinner Date

Meat, bourbon, cupcakes, mmm. This is an all-out (but not difficult) dinner for a man who deserves it. Most evenings, you'll just want to make the steak, mushrooms, and salad—but for special occasions, the whole shebang is spectacular. Besides, we have yet to meet a guy who doesn't like pigs in a blanket for breakfast.

Classic Manhattans with Maraschino Cherries, PAGE 72

Pigs in a Blanket, PAGE 47

Seared Steaks Drizzled with Warm Butter, PAGE 105

Mushrooms Sautéed with Garlic and Red Onion, PAGE 191

Arugula and Grapefruit Salad with Shallot Vinaigrette, PAGE 91

Chocolate and Dark Beer Cupcakes with Irish Cream Frosting, PAGE 227

You Landed Your Dream Job Champagne Brunch

Why wait for someone else to throw you a party? Celebrate yourself! If you're popping open the bubbly (and we encourage you to do so, early and often), you need easy, fast, special dishes like these all-grown-up versions of the breakfast foods you loved as a kid.

Mimosas, PAGE 65

Raspberry-Ricotta Pancakes, PAGE 36

Crisp, Oven-Cooked Bacon with Brown Sugar, PAGE 25

Fabulous Fruit Plate (See Kitchen Basics, PAGE 240)

I Like You Enough to Cook Dinner

You asked him over. You consulted your girls about what to wear. You Swiffered. Now all you have to do is cook him something that shows A) you care, but B) you're not trying too hard. This menu nails it, and won't leave you so tired that you're not up for some fun once the dishes are cleared.

Cucumber Gimlets, PAGE 69

Broiled Baguette Toasts with Assorted Toppings, PAGE 48

Sweet Potato Fries with Crispy Sage, PAGE 195

Tuna Steaks Seared with Ginger, Soy, and Brown Sugar, PAGE 133

Rich, Chocolate Brownies, PAGE 233

Ladies Who Lunch, 2.0

This is not your mother's finger-sandwiches luncheon (although if you invite her, she'll swoon with pride!). Perfect pre-wedding, for a shower, or on any given Sunday, it's just enough food to keep everyone eating and chatting for hours—but not so heavy that you don't have room for cookies.

Bloody Marys, PAGE 66

Lemony White Bean Dip with Arugula, Garlic, and Sea Salt, PAGE 54

Mixed Greens with Roquefort Cheese, Pomegranate, and Rosemary-Lime Dressing, PAGE 88

Chocolate-Chocolate Chip Cookies, PAGE 234

Don't Block the TV Dinner Party

Having people over for the Oscars, the Super Bowl, or, okay, just another reality-show evening? Almost every recipe on this menu can be easily doubled or tripled and made ahead of time. Also, you can eat it all on the couch—no plates required. (Try using mugs for the chili!)

Fresh Homemade Salsa with Tomato, Cilantro, and Jalapeño, PAGE 53

Creamy Artichoke and Cheese Party Dip, PAGE 52

Crusty Grilled Cheese Sandwiches, PAGE 213

Meaty Chili Spiked with Jalapeños and Cheese, PAGE 204

Frosted Vanilla Cupcakes, PAGE 225

Birthday Party for Your BFF

The laughter, the tears, the middle-of-the-night phone calls: She who has stuck with you through the worst deserves the best. Easy Mexican food and a pitcher of margaritas guarantees that what happens at her party stays at her party. (If your crew is small, you can choose either tostadas *or* tacos.)

Pink Watermelon Margaritas, PAGE 67

Spicy Mexican Beer Cockails, PAGE 71

Guacamole with Red Onion, Cilantro, and Lime, PAGE 51

Crunchy Homemade Tostadas with Spicy Beef, Cheddar Cheese, and Fresh Salsa, PAGE 115

Lime Tilapia Fish Tacos, PAGE 206

Vanilla Layer Cake with Chocolate Buttercream Frosting, PAGE 219

Don't Blow Your Diet Dinner with the Girls

Maybe you're trying to live healthfully . . . or maybe your friends are, and you want to do right by them. With a delicious kale salad, elegant salmon, and easy, yummy green beans, this is a meal you'll all feel great after eating. And the best part? Plenty of room for a healthy dessert!

White Sangría, PAGE 73

Caesar-Style Salad with Kale, Pecorino Cheese, and Homemade Croutons, PAGE 89

Salmon with Lemon, White Wine, and Capers, PAGE 134

Gingery Green Beans, PAGE 196

Sweet Mixed Berries with Port, PAGE 237

Come Over for
Drinks and Dessert Party

"Oh, we're all headed to _____'s." Want your place to become that place? No need to cook full three-course meals for the masses. Drinks and sweet treats do the trick every time. And this menu works well both at 4:00 P.M.... and at midnight (brilliant New Year's Eve idea!).

Mojitos, PAGE 68

Tart Strawberry Lemonade, PAGE 74

Perfect Cheese Plate (see Kitchen Basics, PAGE 60)

Fresh-Baked Cobbler with Ripe Plums and Sweet
Buttermilk Crust, PAGE 231

Classic Apple Pie with Buttery Crust, PAGE 229

Chocolate-Chocolate Chip Cookies, PAGE 234

Easy and Elegant Dinner Party

Your own place: check. Plates that aren't paper: check. An excuse to show off both: We've got you covered. It's time to spread those grown-woman wings and host your first simple-yet-chic dinner party. Easy and light dishes like our spiked glazed nuts and Mediterranean-style scallops are sure to impress.

Cucumber Gimlets, PAGE 69

Nuts Spiked with Cinnamon and Cayenne, PAGE 55

Salad of Watermelon, Tomatoes, Mint, and Almonds with Sherry Vinaigrette, PAGE 92

Mediterranean-Style Scallops with Olives and Oregano, PAGE 140

Traditional Italian Affogato, PAGE 235

kitchen basics:

Everything You Need for a Well-Stocked Kitchen

WHAT EVERY WOMAN SHOULD HAVE IN HER PANTRY

The idea of a well-stocked pantry may be intimidating (who even *has* a pantry these days?). But you'll save time—and, even more significantly, the money you would have spent on last-minute purchases—if you keep a few essentials on hand. And consider: If every time you do a big grocery shopping, you add just one or two items on this list, in six months' time you'll be set.

PANTRY

Flour (all-purpose)

Sugar (granulated, confectioners', brown)

Baking soda

Baking powder (always check the expiration date before using; it can lose its efficacy)

Pasta (spaghetti, penne, fusilli, or other favorite kinds)

Rice (long-grain, Arborio, brown)

Couscous

Bread crumbs

Beans (black, pinto, cannellini, garbanzo, kidney)

Olive oil (for cooking) and extra-virgin olive oil (for salads)

Vegetable oil

Cooking spray

Vinegar (Balsamic, red-wine vinegar, sherry)

Whole canned tomatoes (preferably San Marzano)

Chicken broth (or bouillon cubes)

Worcestershire sauce

Soy sauce

Sesame oil

A good mustard (like Dijon)

Canned tuna (preferably packed in olive oil)

Honey
Maple syrup
Jam or jelly
Pure vanilla extract
Capers

Anchovies
Nuts
Raisins
Milk boxes (they're shelf-stable for
    months, in case of emergencies)

HERBS AND SPICES
Sea salt or kosher salt
Iodized salt
Peppercorns
Ground cinnamon
Ground nutmeg
Ground turmeric
Cayenne

Ground ginger
Ground cumin
Paprika
Dried oregano
Dried rosemary
Dried thyme
Bay leaves

THE ONLY TOOLS YOU NEED TO OWN

Do you walk into a shiny kitchenware store and want to snap up everything in sight? We know the feeling—but who can afford *that*? So we've made it easy: Below is a quick checklist for must-have equipment, the stuff that will get you started with maximum flexibility and minimum cost.

For advice, we turned to Lynne Rossetto Kasper and Sally Swift, the host and producer, respectively, of American Public Media's award-winning radio show, *The Splendid Table*. As you build your kitchen, keep Lynne and Sally's theory in mind: "The things you see in your sink the most are the things where you need the best quality you can afford." So the list below is just a guideline; *you* are the expert on what you really need.

As for where to shop, consider ethnic markets or sites like kalustyans.com; Lynne recommends both as sources of good-quality items that are often less than half the usual price.

THE BARE ESSENTIALS

You can make nearly everything in this cookbook with these few items:

- Mixing bowls: Everyone and their mother loves oh-so-durable, freezer-to-oven Pyrex.

- Measuring cups and spoons: For liquid measuring, get one 4-cup measuring cup; for dry measuring, get a set of cups ranging from ¼ to 1 cup.

- Sauce pan: "A 4-quart sauce pan is perfect for your ½ pound of pasta and small stews," says Lynne.

- Colander: Use to wash fruits or vegetables, strain ingredients, and drain pasta.

- 12-inch frying pan: A cast-iron pan is an inexpensive, sturdy alternative to stainless steel. Whatever material you get, make sure the pan has a metal handle, not wood or plastic, says Sally and Lynne. With that, you can roast a chicken in the oven, grill burgers when it's too cold out, make a casserole—it's the everything pan, and you can live on that!

- Baking pan: A sheet of thick aluminum with rolled edges that is as big as your oven is mighty handy: Right-side up, it's the perfect tool to roast vegetables; flip it upside down, and it's a huge cookie sheet. And thick aluminum won't bend or warp.

- Spatula: Consider getting a combination spoon-spatula with a straight edge; Lynne swears these cheap tools do twice the work with half the effort.

- Heavy-duty tongs: "I use tongs for everything," says Sally. "With long-handled tongs, you can roast peppers, pull pans out of the oven, grab things under the couch . . ."

- Knives: "Ethnic markets have baskets full of cheap, ceramic paring knives," says Sally. Get the ones with their own slipcovers, so they don't bang around and chip in your drawers (or cut your fingers when you reach in!).

- Kitchen towels: Kitchen towels are cheaper and more versatile than hot pads or oven mitts—Ikea sells great ones for almost nothing.

- Spoons: Lynne and Sally recommend two—a big stainless-steel spoon for tasting sauces, and a slotted spoon—both dishwasher-safe and usually quite inexpensive.

- Cutting board: A must to protect your counters.

- Corkscrew: A *Glamour*-girl essential—need we say more?

NEXT STEPS

When you're more comfy in your kitchen and looking to expand, consider:

- Covered Dutch oven: Sally says she uses her cast-iron, 6-quart Dutch oven more than anything else in her kitchen. It would work perfectly for beefy, meaty meals, like our Single Digit Grocery Bill Stew or It's Almost Payday Chili.

- Blender

- Wok: Find a rolled steel or cast-iron Chinese wok with a flat bottom and wooden handle. It's not just for stir-fry; you can boil sauce, fry eggs, make mac and cheese, *anything*.

AFFORDABLE ADD-ONS

Collect these piece by piece:

- Whisk

- Peeler

- Meat thermometer

- Pepper grinder

- Offset spatula (the thin metal kind, good for working with frosting or pastry crust)

- Grater

- Potato masher

- Salad spinner

BIT OF A SPLURGE

You can ask for these as presents (or treat yourself):

- Immersion blender (the hand-held kind that blends foods in the pan or bowl)

- Toaster oven

- Mortar and pestle

FINAL ACQUISITIONS

- Food processor

- Chef's knife (or a whole set of knives, in a block): Make sure it feels comfortable in your hand and has an 8-inch blade that runs through the handle. Keep it sharp with slipcovers or invest in a wooden knife block.

- Full set of good-quality pots and pans: These don't have to break the bank, and as you get more proficient you're going to want a variety of sizes, with lids.

Acknowledgments

WHEN IT COMES TO CREATING A GOOD COOKBOOK, THERE IS no such thing as too many cooks in the kitchen. This book is the brainchild of *dozens* of such cooks: *Glamour* editors over the generations who have created and published recipes with women's real lives in mind.

Glamour contributing editor Kimberly Bonnell got the ball rolling with her original Engagement Chicken recipe. We, and 60-plus couples, thank her. Cookbook editor Veronica Chambers then shaped this collection, wrestling with tricky decisions about which recipes should make the cut, and weaving the 100 that did into a cohesive, satisfying book. Contributing cookbook editors Salma Abdelnour and Erin Zammett Ruddy updated many recipes, integrating feedback from readers and recipe testers, and rolling up their sleeves in their own kitchens. *Glamour* editorial development director Susan Goodall organized the entire project with chef-like efficiency, and assistant editor Carly Suber kept all the details in line. On the design side, *Glamour* design director Geraldine Hessler lent her unerring sense of style, and senior photo editor Martha Maristany conceived and produced the photos that open and close the book. Copy editor Lene Dahl and researcher Penny Wrenn polished the manuscript, and former *Glamour* executive editor Jill Herzig helped shape the book in its early stages. We're grateful for the enthusiasm and support of our partners at Hyperion, especially president and publisher Ellen Archer, who championed this project, and editor in chief Elisabeth Dyssegaard, who helped make it sing. Special thanks to literary agent David Kuhn, who shares our belief in the power of a good meal—including the lunch of Dover sole and salad over which the idea for this cookbook was hatched.

Back to all those cooks in the kitchen. Thanks goes to the extended *Glamour* family members who tried out all the recipes in kitchens big and small: Ranya Barrett, Lauren Brody, Brittany Burke, Ayana Byrd, Caroline Campion, Jessica Duncan, Troy Dunham, Jenny Feldman, Linda Fiorella, Mari Gill, Amanda Grooms West, William Hooks, Sarah Jio, Amber Kallor, Brian Marcus, Kaitlin Menza, Eilish Morley, Baze Mpinja, Joanna Muenz, Wendy Naugle, Leslie Robarge, Anne Sachs, Laura Smith, Jessica Strul, Meredith Turits, and Lindsey Unterberger. And thanks especially to the experienced recipe testers who double-checked each recipe, adjusting and re-imagining ingredients when necessary: Paul Grimes, Gina Marie Miraglia Eriquez, Marisa Robertson-Textor, and Shelley Wiseman.

Glamour would also like to thank: Shubhani Sarkar, Navorn Johnson, Suzanne Donaldson, Noah Dreier, Sarah Viñas, Theresa Griggs, Diane Morgan, Lynne Rossetto Kasper, Sally Swift, Patrick Fusco, Jeff Mikkelson, Hillary Seitz, Charlie Palmer, Andrew Weil, Marcus Samuelsson, Klancy Miller, Vickie Myers, Laura Wheeler, Bernadette Anat, Jamie Bachmann, Megan Baker, Elizabeth Kreutz, and Alison Goldman.

And most of all, thanks to *you*, the woman holding this book in her hands. Without the stories you tell us every month—about the dishes you make, and the magic that happens along the way—our jobs would not be half as delicious.

Index

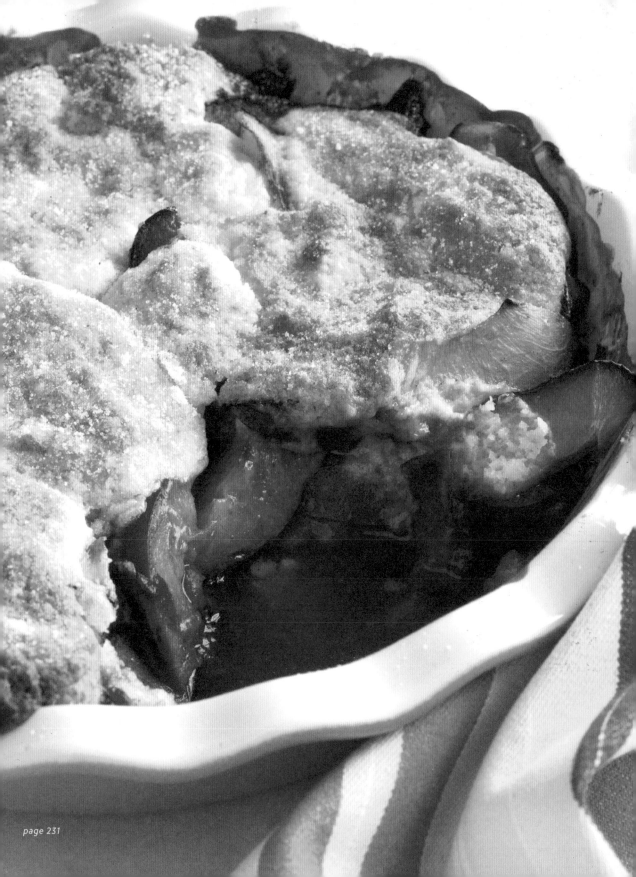